Behavioral Addictions

Behavioral Addictions

DSM-5® and Beyond

EDITED BY NANCY M. PETRY

OXFORD
UNIVERSITY PRESS

Oxford University Press is a department of the University of
Oxford. It furthers the University's objective of excellence in research,
scholarship, and education by publishing worldwide.

Oxford   New York
Auckland   Cape Town   Dar es Salaam   Hong Kong   Karachi
Kuala Lumpur   Madrid   Melbourne   Mexico City   Nairobi
New Delhi   Shanghai   Taipei   Toronto

With offices in
Argentina   Austria   Brazil   Chile   Czech Republic   France   Greece
Guatemala   Hungary   Italy   Japan   Poland   Portugal   Singapore
South Korea   Switzerland   Thailand   Turkey   Ukraine   Vietnam

Published in the United States of America by
Oxford University Press
198 Madison Avenue, New York, NY 10016

Cataloging-in-Publication data is on file at the Library of Congress
ISBN 978-0-19-939154-7

The Diagnostic and Statistical Manual of Mental Disorders, DSM, DSM-IV, DSM-IV-TR, and
DSM-5 are registered trademarks of the American Psychiatric Association. Oxford University Press
USA is not associated with the American Psychiatric Association or with any of its products or
publications, nor do the views expressed herein represent the policies and opinions of the American
Psychiatric Association.

9 8 7 6 5 4 3 2
Printed in Canada
on acid-free paper

For Billy, Hannah, and Noah

CONTENTS

CONTRIBUTORS

Nicole M. Avena, PhD
Department of Pharmacology
 and Systems Therapeutics
Mount Sinai School of Medicine
New York, NY

Donald W. Black, PhD
Department of Psychiatry
University of Iowa Roy J.
 and Lucille A. Carver College
 of Medicine
Iowa City, IA

Megan M. Campbell, PhD
Department of Psychiatry
 and Mental Health
University of Cape Town
Cape Town, South Africa

Elliot J. Coups, PhD
Rutgers Cancer Institute
 of New Jersey
Rutgers, The State University
 of New Jersey
New Brunswick, NJ

Mark S. Gold, MD
Department of Psychiatry
Washington University School
 of Medicine
St. Louis, MO

Joel Hillhouse, PhD
East Tennessee State University
Johnson City, TN

Simone Kühn, PhD
Max Planck Institute for Human
 Development
Center for Lifespan Psychology
Berlin, Germany
University Clinic
 Hamburg-Eppendorf
Clinic and Policlinic for Psychiatry
 and Psychotherapy
Hamburg, Germany

Susan Murray, BS
Department of Pharmacology
 and Systems Therapeutics
Mount Sinai School of Medicine
New York, NY

Nancy M. Petry, PhD
Department of Medicine
   and Calhoun Cardiology Center
University of Connecticut School
   of Medicine
Farmington, CT

Florian Rehbein, PhD
Criminological Research Institute
   of Lower Saxony
Hanover, Germany

Hans-Jürgen Rumpf, PD Dipl Psych
Department of Psychiatry
   and Psychotherapy
University of Lübeck
Lübeck, Germany

Jerod L. Stapleton, PhD
Rutgers Cancer Institute of
   New Jersey
Rutgers, The State University
   of New Jersey
New Brunswick, NJ

Dan J. Stein, MD, PhD
Professor and Chair
Department of Psychiatry
University of Cape Town
Cape Town, South Africa

Ran Tao
Addiction Medical Center
General Hospital of Beijing
      Military Region
Beijing, China

Aviv Weinstein, PhD
Department of Behavioral Science
University of Ariel
Ariel, Israel

Yitzhak Weinstein, PhD
Ohalo Academic College
College Park, Israel
Tel Hai Academic College
Tel-Hai, Israel
Israel Institute of Technology
Haifa, Israel

Introduction to Behavioral Addictions

NANCY M. PETRY ■

The concept of behavioral addiction has been a topic of debate for decades. Research and clinical experiences suggest that behaviors that occur in extremes can result in substantial problems, regardless of the nature of the specific activity. People can smoke cigarettes, drink alcohol, use drugs, gamble, play video games, use the Internet, engage in sexual activities, shop, exercise, eat, or tan to excess. Growing evidence indicates that extensive, repetitive, and problematic engagement in these activities can share some similarities with substance use disorders. Overlap may exist in terms of phenomenology (craving, tolerance, and withdrawal), natural history (onset, chronicity, and relapsing course), comorbidity, genetic overlap and neurobiological mechanisms, and response to treatment. As the behaviors increase in frequency and duration, they can lead to psychological distress and sometimes even physical impairment, as well as diminish social, financial, and occupational functioning.

Addiction, however, is a loaded term. It has different meanings to different people. Colloquially, it refers to excessive use of a substance or participation in a behavior. Clinically, it can signify loss of control and impairment in functioning. Substance use disorders are often called "addictions," and they have been recognized as psychiatric diseases for decades. Some have argued against the term "addiction" in this context because it can have pejorative and nonmedical meanings. Others contend that the term appropriately refers to the nature in which individuals with substance use disorders consume alcohol and drugs and develop difficulties with other behaviors as well.

In 2013, the publication of the fifth revision of the *Diagnostic and Statistical Manual of Mental Disorders* (DSM-5) opened the door for classification of non-substance addictions—that is, behavioral addictions. The DSM is the primary psychiatric diagnostic classification system in the United States, and clinicians and researchers in many other countries throughout the world apply it as well. For the first time, this manual recognizes behavioral addictions.

Although the DSM-5 does not officially term substance use disorders "addictions," the chapter containing them broadened these conditions to "Substance-Related and Addictive Disorders." This chapter now lists substance use disorders, such as alcohol, opioids, stimulants, cannabis, nicotine, hallucinogens, inhalant, and sedatives, along with one non-substance or behavioral addiction—gambling disorder (Chapter 2).

Formerly termed "pathological gambling," the DSM has included a condition related to excessive and problematic gambling since 1980. With publication of DSM-III and throughout the next 33 years, pathological gambling was a Disorder of Impulse Control Disorder Not Elsewhere Classified. The most recent version of the DSM altered the name to "gambling disorder" and moved it alongside substance use disorders as the first non-substance or behavioral addiction. This change opens the possibility for classifications of other excessive behavior patterns as addictions as well.

Although some researchers and clinicians support expansion of addictions as a construct, proliferation of psychiatric conditions can diminish the legitimacy of the field of psychiatry at large. It is important to distinguish true mental disorders from high levels of normal behavior patterns. Surely not everyone should have a psychiatric condition, and if many excessive behavioral patterns are deemed psychiatric disorders most everyone would be diagnosed with mental illness. This concern is particularly relevant to the construct of behavioral addictions. Excessive chocolate eating, even if it is causing weight gain and some distress, does not constitute a psychiatric disorder.

In preparing for the DSM-5, researchers and clinicians considered many putative non-substance addictions for inclusion in the manual. Workgroup members formed specialized subcommittees composed of experts in specific areas. They reviewed existing literature and made recommendations regarding whether there was sufficient evidence to propose new disorders for inclusion in the DSM-5.

Introduction of a new psychiatric diagnosis in the DSM-5 required scientific evidence, confirmed by expert consensus. Clinicians and researchers both within and disparate from the specific clinical area reviewed the data and arguments presented and voted on whether or not data were sufficiently strong to include new conditions in the DSM-5. Prior to official voting, the workgroups posted online recommendations for changes to existing disorders and proposals for new disorders, and other clinicians, researchers, and the public at large could comment on these suggestions during two open commentary periods.

The American Psychiatric Association noted that newly included disorders must fulfill a clinical need, reflect an underlying psychobiological disturbance, and contribute to better assessment and treatment. At the most basic level, psychiatric disorders must engender clinically significant harm, and not merely reflect social deviance or conflicts with society. New conditions also had to be sufficiently distinct from existing disorders. Although comorbidity may be high, a newly introduced disorder must be distinguishable from existing ones to be uniquely classified. It must have diagnostic validity, and data must be available indicating that the proposed criteria reliably and validly classify individuals with the condition. The DSM-5 added only 15 disorders that were not contained in the DSM-IV. None were behavioral addictions.

Although no new diagnoses related to behavioral addictions appear in the DSM-5, Section 3, the research appendix, includes one. The intent of this section is to stimulate research on conditions that may be psychiatric disorders but for which sufficient data do not yet exist to reliably and validly classify them. Based on the available published literature through 2012, one behavioral addiction was deemed to have sufficient data to warrant its inclusion in the research appendix—Internet gaming disorder (Chapter 3).

Workgroup members and the scientific community at large considered other behavioral addictions as well: Internet addiction (Chapter 4), sex addiction (Chapter 5), shopping addiction (Chapter 6), exercise addiction (Chapter 7), eating addiction (Chapter 8), and tanning addiction (Chapter 9). This book describes each of these putative behavioral addictions. The chapters outline the existing research related to each condition, and they also provide rationale as to why the data were not yet sufficient to include them in the DSM-5.

Although these other conditions are not officially recognized in the DSM-5, this does not mean they are not psychiatric disorders. Their lack of inclusion simply reflects a lack of scientific evidence related to diagnostic assessment, clinical course, or treatment. As described in the subsequent eight chapters in this book, some have more, and some fewer, scientific data related to their uniqueness as a psychiatric disorder and along these dimensions. As science progresses, subsequent versions of the DSM may officially classify some of them as psychiatric conditions. Until then, these chapters provide state-of-the-art reviews of the scientific data surrounding each.

The chapters begin with a global overview of the condition and its actual or proposed diagnostic criteria. The chapters next outline the various instruments designed to assess each condition and their psychometric properties. Prevalence rates in general populations and specific and clinical populations are detailed. In addition, comorbidities with substance use and other psychiatric conditions are described. The chapters also review the risk and protective factors related to each condition, including the biological and genetic data that exist. A section of each chapter reviews treatments found efficacious in randomized trials or applied clinically when no or few randomized clinical trials exist. Finally, each chapter summarizes strengths and limitations of the existing data related to the condition. For all except gambling disorders, the chapters specify areas in which additional research is needed for their potential classification and recognition as unique psychiatric disorders in future editions of the DSM. Together, these chapters provide a comprehensive and timely scientific review of behavioral addictions. They should be valuable for guiding future research, and clinical care, across behavioral addictions.

2

Gambling Disorder

The First Officially Recognized Behavioral Addiction

NANCY M. PETRY ◼

Gambling disorder, previously termed pathological gambling, is the first disorder to be included as a non-substance behavioral addiction in the fifth edition of the *Diagnostic and Statistical Manual of Mental Disorders* (DSM-5; American Psychiatric Association, 2013). This chapter outlines the DSM-5 classification system for gambling disorder and instruments that assess it. It details the prevalence rates in the general population of the United States as well as in other countries throughout the world. The chapter also describes comorbidities between gambling disorder and other psychiatric conditions, focusing on its overlap with substance use disorders. The risk and protective factors are then outlined, including demographic, psychological, neurophysiological, and genetic risk factors. Finally, the chapter summarizes both promising psychological and pharmacological treatments and discusses future research directions to improve the diagnosis, prevention, and treatment of this behavioral addiction.

DEFINING FEATURES AND METHODS FOR ASSESSMENT

Gambling disorder is the first "behavioral addiction" listed in the DSM. The DSM has included gambling disorder, previously termed "pathological gambling" since 1980. However, it was classified as an "Impulse

Control Disorder Not Otherwise Specified" until the publication of the DSM-5. Given considerable overlap between gambling and substance use disorders (Petry et al., 2013), it is now included in the "Substance Use and Related Addictive Disorders" section.

The DSM-5 lists nine criteria, and for a diagnosis one must endorse at least four of the following: (1) spending a lot of time thinking about gambling or where to get money with which to gamble (i.e., "preoccupation"), (2) needing to wager with larger amounts (i.e., tolerance), (3) repeated unsuccessful attempts to stop or control gambling, (4) experiencing withdrawal symptoms such as restlessness or irritability when trying to cease or reduce gambling, (5) wagering to escape from problems or to relieve negative moods, (6) trying to recoup prior gambling losses (i.e., "chasing"), (7) lying to others about one's gambling or trying to cover up the extent of gambling, (8) losing relationships or a career or educational opportunity due to gambling, and (9) relying on others to relieve a desperate financial situation caused by gambling (i.e., "bailouts"). Although not a diagnosed psychiatric condition, problem gambling is a term used to describe meeting less than the requisite number of DSM criteria for diagnosis.

Structured clinical interviews, employing these DSM criteria, can diagnose gambling disorder or classify individuals as problem gamblers. One structured clinical interview that assesses gambling disorder criteria is the Alcohol Use Disorder and Associated Disabilities Interview Schedule–DSM-IV Version (AUDASIS). It contains 15 items, with one or two symptoms constituting each of the DSM criteria for gambling disorder; if respondents endorse either or both items associated with a criterion, they meet that criterion. Internal consistency of the items and test–retest reliability are excellent (Grant et al., 2003; Petry et al., 2005).

Another structured clinical interview is the National Opinion Research Center DSM-IV Screen for Gambling Problems or NODS (Gerstein et al., 1999). This instrument also assesses DSM gambling symptoms, again using one or two items per criterion, although the specific wording of the items differs from that of the AUDASIS. The test–retest reliability of the

NODS is excellent (Gerstein et al., 1999), and validity is well established in multiple samples (Hodgins, 2004; Petry, 2007; Wickwire et al., 2008; Wulfert et al., 2005).

The AUDASIS and NODS are the most common diagnostic instruments for gambling disorders. The Canadian Problem Gambling Severity Index (PGSI) is popular in Canada, and some other countries have begun using this instrument as well. The PGSI contains nine items, but the items are not aligned, or intended to relate directly, to the DSM-5 criteria for gambling disorder. Instead, the items reflect more socially oriented (rather than clinical) aspects of problem gambling. The nine items are rated on a 4-point scale with total scores ranging from 0 to 27. Score on the PGSI correlate with other DSM-based scales such as the NODS (Ferris and Wynne, 2001). Individuals who score 0 are termed "non-problem gamblers," and categories of increasing risk range from "low-risk" to "moderate risk" and "problem gamblers," depending on scale scores (Ferris and Wynne, 2001). Although numerous studies have applied this instrument, some have raised concerns about the nature of the scoring system and validity of the classification structure. For example, Orford et al. (2010) compared the PGSI and a DSM-IV scale using data from 6,161 adult past-year gamblers in the United Kingdom. Although the PGSI had good internal reliability, the rate of agreement between the two instruments for identifying individuals with gambling problems was only modest, and there was evidence that the PGSI may underestimate gambling problems, particularly in women. Currie et al. (2013) likewise noted potential problems with the scale. The temporal stability was adequate during a 14-month interval, but the four proposed categories of gamblers were not well discriminated. Currie et al. suggested the instrument would benefit from changes in the scoring system and greater psychometric testing, especially for the at-risk problem gambling classifications.

The South Oaks Gambling Screen (SOGS; Lesieur and Blume, 1987), similar to the PGSI, is a screener for gambling problems and not designed to provide diagnoses. It is the oldest and most commonly applied screening instrument, and it has been translated into approximately two dozen languages. This 20-item instrument reflects older, DSM-III-R criteria for gambling, with an emphasis on assessing financial problems related to gambling. Scores range from 0 to 20, with scores of 5 or higher typically indicating probable gambling disorder. Because this is a screening instrument, however, it like the PGSI, does not yield diagnoses, and additional assessment is needed to classify individuals with gambling disorder. Furthermore, the SOGS has a high false-positive rate (Stinchfield, 2002), meaning that a fairly large proportion of persons who score high on the SOGS do not meet DSM criteria for gambling disorder. Whereas the SOGS and PGSI are appropriate for assessing risk, if psychiatric diagnosis is desired, one must administer a DSM-based instrument.

Other briefer screening instruments also exist, but limited information about their psychometric properties is available (for review, see Volberg et al., 2011). Perhaps the most promising involve abbreviated versions of the NODS. Toce-Gerstein et al. (2009) compared diagnostic status derived from the 17-item NODS to shorter versions using subsets of 2 to 4 of the NODS items in 8,867 gamblers participating in general population surveys. The three questions pertaining to loss of Control, Lying, and Preoccupation (the NODS-CLiP) identified the vast majority of individuals with gambling disorder diagnosed by the full NODS, with excellent sensitivity and specificity. A follow-up study (Volberg et al., 2011) conducted in high-risk populations (e.g., substance abuse treatment patients and inner-city medical patients) found that some different NODS items yielded the greatest diagnostic accuracy, with positive endorsement of the Preoccupation, Escape, Risked Relationships, and Chasing items best aligning with the full NODS diagnosis. Although the specific items may differ depending on the populations assessed, a two-stage procedure may efficiently identify and then confirm diagnosis of gambling disorder for research studies or clinical practice settings in which inclusion of a full gambling diagnosis interview for all respondents or patients would be burdensome.

Another approach to avoid lengthy questionnaire administration to individuals unlikely to experience gambling problems is to initially inquire about minimal levels of gambling participation prior to administration of a full battery. Epidemiological studies asked gambling disorder criteria only to individuals who reported gambling a nominal number of times (e.g., five times) in their lives (e.g., Gerstein et al., 1999; Petry et al., 2005). Such "gatekeeper" questions, however, should include very minimum participation histories to avoid missing diagnoses. The diagnostic criteria for gambling disorder, similar to those for substance use disorders, do not involve indices of frequency of gambling or amounts wagered. Although frequency and quantity indices relate to harms experienced from gambling, they are not synonymous. For example, some individuals place bets daily, such as scratch ticket players or lottery players, but do not suffer from any gambling-related harm. Financially secure individuals may place very large bets without experiencing any adverse effects, whereas individuals with low and fixed incomes may place relatively small bets but report severe consequences from their gambling (Petry, 2003). Similarly, one person can drink daily without developing alcohol problems, and another binge drinks only occasionally but suffers severe consequences. Although many screening instruments and diagnostic interviews inquire about frequency and quantity of gambling, these indices do not factor into diagnoses.

PREVALENCE RATES

Using the previously described instruments, nationally representative studies of the prevalence rate of gambling disorder have been conducted in the United States. Other countries, including Canada, the United Kingdom, Australia, New Zealand, China, Singapore, Italy, Norway, Sweden, and Switzerland, have also evaluated rates of gambling disorder in national samples. Although prevalence rates vary depending on the time frame of assessment and the instrument applied, most surveys reveal that gambling disorder impacts between 0.1% and 2% of the population.

In the late 1990s, the U.S. government commissioned the National Gambling Impact Study Commission (Gerstein et al., 1999). This study surveyed 2,417 randomly selected U.S. adult residents, using the NODS to assess gambling disorder. It found that the lifetime prevalence rate of gambling disorder was 0.8%, and the past-year prevalence rate was 0.1%. Another nationally based telephone survey of 2,638 randomly selected U.S. adults was conducted at approximately the same time (Welte et al., 2001). Using the SOGS and another instrument based on DSM criteria, it found a higher lifetime prevalence rate of approximately 2.0% for gambling disorder.

Two larger nationally based U.S. surveys of gambling disorder were completed more recently. The National Epidemiologic Survey on Alcohol and Related Conditions (NESARC) conducted in-person interviews with more than 43,000 randomly selected adults. It estimated a lifetime prevalence rate of gambling disorder of 0.4% (Petry et al., 2005) and a past-year prevalence rate of 0.2% (Petry et al., 2013). The National Comorbidity Survey–Replication (NCS-R), composed of 9,282 respondents, likewise found a lifetime prevalence rate of gambling disorder of 0.6%. In this survey, the past-year prevalence rate was 0.3% (Kessler et al., 2008).

Other countries have conducted nationally representative epidemiological surveys as well. Two independent studies in Norway found gambling disorder impacted approximately 0.2% of the population (Gotestam and Johansson, 2003; Lund and Nordlund, 2003). Abbott and Volberg (2000) found that the prevalence rate of gambling disorder was 0.5% in New Zealand; Volberg et al. (2001) found a rate of 0.6% in Sweden; and Orford et al. (2003) and Bondolfi et al. (2000) found rates of 0.8% in the United Kingdom and Switzerland, respectively. The Australian Institute for Gambling Research reported one of the highest rates of gambling disorder in a primarily English-speaking country of 1.9%, but that rate was derived from the SOGS, which tends to overestimate prevalence rates. Using DSM-based criteria, two surveys from Asian countries reported high rates of gambling disorder as well. The Ministry of Community Development (2005) in Singapore and Wong and So (2003) in Hong Kong found rates of 2.1% and 1.8%, respectively. Thus, overall, prevalence rates for gambling disorder in countries throughout the world appear similar to those reported in the United States. A meta-analysis estimated the prevalence rate of gambling disorder to be between 0.8% and 1.8% (Stucki and Rihs-Middel, 2007).

COMORBIDITIES

Gambling disorder is highly comorbid with other psychiatric conditions, especially substance use disorders. Epidemiological studies provide the best evidence of comorbidities, and all published general population surveys evaluating both gambling and substance use disorders found significant associations between them. For example, the National Gambling Impact Survey (Gerstein et al., 1999) found that 9.9% of respondents with gambling disorder met criteria for an alcohol or illicit drug use disorder. In contrast, only 1.1% of non-gamblers and 1.3% of recreational non-problem gamblers had a substance use diagnosis. In the NCS-R survey, Kessler et al. (2008) reported that rates of substance use disorders were 5.5-fold higher among respondents with a gambling disorder compared to those without, and 76.3% of individuals with gambling disorder also had a substance use disorder. Similarly, the NESARC study (Petry et al., 2005) noted a strong association between gambling disorder and substance use disorders. Almost half (47.8%) of individuals identified with gambling disorder also met criteria for alcohol dependence, and more than one-third had one or more other substance use disorder, such as sedative, tranquilizer, opiate, stimulant, hallucinogen, cannabis, cocaine, inhalant/solvent, or heroin use disorder. In contrast, only 8.8% of non-gamblers had an illicit drug use disorder. Surveys from other studies report similar results. In a Canadian survey of 14,934 persons, el-Guebaly et al. (2006) found that nearly half of those identified with gambling problems had substance dependence or harmful use of alcohol versus 7.6% of non-problem gamblers.

Rates of comorbidities with other non-addictive psychiatric disorders are also high. The NESARC study (Petry et al., 2005) found that rates of major depression and dysthymia were approximately three times higher in individuals with gambling disorder than in non-gamblers. Likewise, the NCS-R study (Kessler et al., 2008) reported major depressive disorder or dysthymia to be 2.5 times higher in respondents with gambling disorder compared to respondents without. In terms of anxiety disorders, the NESARC survey found that prevalence rates of every anxiety disorder assessed were significantly elevated among those with gambling disorder compared to those without gambling disorder, including generalized anxiety disorder, panic disorder with and without agoraphobia, specific phobias, and social phobia (Petry et al., 2005). The NCS-R (Kessler et al., 2008) also noted significantly increased rates of panic disorder, phobias, and generalized anxiety disorder in those with gambling disorder compared to those without.

A meta-analysis evaluated the co-occurrence of gambling and other psychiatric conditions in epidemiological surveys conducted in countries throughout the world (Lorains et al., 2011). Despite heterogeneity across studies, gambling disorder was significantly related to nicotine, substance use, mood, and anxiety disorders. The weighted mean proportions of individuals with gambling disorder experiencing each of these other conditions was 60.2%, 57.5%, 37.9% and 37.4%, respectively. Furthermore, Rush et al. (2008) evaluated the association between substance use disorders, other mental health conditions, and gambling problems. Severity of gambling problems increased with severity of substance use problems, but this pattern did not occur with other mental health disorders, and other conditions did not impact the relationship between gambling and substance use problems. In summary, strong and consistent relationships exist between gambling disorder and other psychiatric disorders, but these associations appear strongest with substance use disorders.

The relationships between gambling disorder and other behavioral addictions are not yet well understood, in part because there are few large-scale epidemiological surveys of other behavioral addictions. Most of those that exist did not assess other psychiatric disorders. Nevertheless, available data suggest a relationship between gambling and some other behavioral addictions in adolescents. For example, in an Italian sample of 2,853 high school students, Villella et al. (2011) found that severity of gambling problems was positively associated with severity of problems of other putative behavioral addictions, including exercise, Internet, work, and excessive shopping. In a sample of 1,012 students in Switzerland, Tozzi et al. (2013) found that problem gambling was related to substance use as well as Internet addiction problems. Delfabbro et al. (2009) evaluated the relationship between video game playing and gambling disorder in 2,669 adolescents. Frequency of video game playing was significantly, albeit modestly, correlated with gambling disorder. Similarly, Walther et al. (2012) collected data from 2,553 German students aged 12–25 years and found a small but significant association between gambling and gaming problems. In a sample of more than 73,000 Korean youth, both smoking and drug use were significantly related to Internet addiction problems (Lee et al., 2013). Thus, gambling disorder appears to relate to other behavioral addictions, but the available data are relatively limited and primarily restricted to youth and young adults.

RISK AND PROTECTIVE FACTORS

Demographic Correlates

Some demographic characteristics are associated with gambling disorder, including gender, age, socioeconomic status, and race/ethnicity. Males have an increased risk of gambling problems relative to females. For example, in the NESARC survey (Petry et al., 2005), although the sample was half male and half female, 72% of the individuals classified with gambling disorder were male. Likewise, in the NCS-R (Kessler et al., 2008), men had a 4.5-fold increased risk of developing gambling disorder compared to women. However, data from this survey also revealed that this gender differential may relate to a greater propensity to gamble in men. Men were significantly more likely than women to report having ever gambled, but men who had gambled were no more likely than women who had gambled to develop a gambling problem or to progress from problem gambling to gambling disorder once they began wagering.

Age is inversely associated with gambling disorder in most epidemiological surveys. For example, in the NCS-R survey (Kessler et al., 2008),
respondents in the 18- to 44-year-old cohort had a fivefold increased risk
of developing gambling disorder relative to cohorts older than age 45 years.
The National Gambling Impact Study (Gerstein et al., 1999) likewise found
that the youngest age groups had an increased rate of gambling disorder
relative to the older age group. However, most nationally representative
studies include only individuals aged 18 years or older. Studies restricted
to adolescent and young adults generally find high rates of gambling disorder (Petry, 2005), but assessment instruments for youth often vary from
those for adults (Stinchfield, 2010), as do sampling procedures and survey
designs (Volberg et al., 2010); thus, differences in prevalence rates may be
confounded by differences in methods of assessment. Nevertheless, gambling disorder is typically more prevalent in younger age groups.

In most industrialized countries, gambling disorder is more common
in individuals of racial and ethnic minority backgrounds. For example,
in the U.S. surveys, gambling disorder is more prevalent in African
Americans than it is among European Americans (Kessler et al., 2008;
Petry et al., 2005; Welte et al., 2001). Furthermore, in Canada as well as
the United States, very high rates of gambling problems and gambling
disorder occur in Native Americans as well as in Asian Americans (Petry
et al., 2003; Wardman et al., 2001).

Lower socioeconomic status, which is typically linked with minority
status, is also associated with gambling disorder. Most studies show that
individuals with lower incomes or education are overrepresented among
those with gambling disorder (e.g., Gerstein et al., 1999; Kessler et al.,
2008; Welte et al., 2001).

Personality Factors

In addition to these basic demographic characteristics, impulsivity is
a strong and consistent personality risk factor for gambling disorder.
Impulsivity is a multifaceted construct, involving inattention, disinhibition,

risk-taking, sensation seeking, and discounting of delayed and probabilistic outcomes (Evenden, 1999). In cross-sectional studies, those with gambling disorder evidence increased impulsivity, assessed in a variety of manners, compared to controls (van Holst et al., 2010). Likewise, behavioral and personality measures of impulsivity are higher in substance abusing populations than in controls (Verdejo-Garcia et al., 2008), with data indicating that dual addictive problems (e.g., both substance abuse and gambling disorders) have additive effects on impulsivity (Petry, 2001; Petry and Casarella, 1999).

Furthermore, prospective studies demonstrate that impulsivity in childhood can predict later development of gambling problems (Pagani et al., 2009; Slutske et al., 2012; Vitaro et al., 1999). Likewise, measures of impulsivity and behavioral disinhibition collected from early childhood onward predict later onset of substance use and substance use disorders (Chassin et al., 2004; Guo et al., 2001; Hawkins et al., 1992; Hill et al., 2000; Kandel et al., 1978; McGue et al., 1997; Sher et al., 2000; Zucker, 2008), suggesting a common link between impulsivity and addictive disorders (Slutske et al., 2005).

Neurobiological Risk Factors

In concert with the associations between impulsivity and addictive disorders, studies have demonstrated some similarities between individuals with gambling and substance use disorders in terms of impaired functioning in brain regions that relate to impulsive decision-making and motivational processes more generally. Drugs of abuse increase dopamine transmission on motivational circuits in the brain, including the striatum and the medial prefrontal cortex (PFC; Wise, 2004), and it is primarily in these reward and decision areas that differences are noted in individuals with gambling disorder compared to controls.

The reward deficiency hypothesis predicts that susceptibility to addiction stems from an insensitive dopamine system. According to this theory, individuals with a hypoactive reward system require stronger stimuli (e.g., drugs and gambling) to activate reward systems. In support of this theory, positron emission tomography studies indicate that addicted individuals release less dopamine in response to drug administration than do controls (Martinez et al., 2007; Volkow et al., 1997), and reduced dopamine receptor density in the striatum has been associated with addiction to numerous substances (Volkow et al., 1996, 2001). In functional magnetic resonance imaging studies, however, data are mixed (Hommer et al., 2011). Some studies find a lower striatal response during reward anticipation tasks in substance users relative to controls (Peters et al., 2011), and others report enhanced responses (Jia et al., 2011). Different results may relate to variations in demographic or clinical factors of participants, as well as tasks. In addition, in the case of substance use disorders, it is not clear whether continued use of the substance alters brain structure and functioning or whether deficits precede the onset of substance use disorders.

Studying non-substance addictions, such as gambling, provides a method to tease apart direct effects of substances on the brain from structural and functional impairment. Although gambling may engender neuroadaptive changes in the brain, studies of patients with gambling disorder reveal no gross structural abnormalities in gray or white matter volume (Joutsa et al., 2011; van Holst et al., 2012a). In terms of functional impairment, one of the earliest studies in gamblers found that signal change in the ventral striatum and ventral medial PFC was reduced in individuals with gambling disorder compared to controls and correlated with the severity of gambling symptoms (Reuter et al., 2005). Balodis et al. (2012) also reported a reduction in response to rewards in the ventral striatum among individuals with gambling disorder, but van Holst et al. (2012b) found that gamblers emitted greater response to rewards in the dorsal striatum compared to controls. Variations in tasks may explain some of these differences, with data suggesting that gamblers are particularly sensitive to high-risk rewards. For example, Miedl et al. (2010) found no differences between gamblers and controls during presentation of low-risk rewards, whereas enhanced inferior frontal gyrus and thalamus activity occurred with high-risk rewards. Sescousse et al. (2010) found that individuals with gambling disorder had reduced neural responses to non-gambling and non-monetary rewards in the ventral striatum compared to controls, and these results were consistent with those of individuals with cocaine use disorder (Asensio et al., 2010). However, when the reward was monetary, gamblers demonstrated an increased response in the orbitofrontal cortex relative to controls (Sescousse et al., 2010). In another study, Miedl et al. (2012) found that compared to controls, individuals with gambling disorder showed greater responses in the ventral striatum during temporal discounting of rewards but reduced response during probabilistic discounting. Given these complexities and differences across reward types and magnitudes, it is unclear to what extent substance use and gambling disorder represent overlapping or distinct frontostriatal dysregulation. To uncover the neurobiology underlying addictive behaviors, future research should employ similar paradigms and tasks across populations to best understand similarities and differences of addictions.

Genetics

Early studies demonstrated that gambling disorder tends to run in families. In community samples, adults identified with gambling disorder are more likely than those without to report having a parent with gambling problems (Volberg and Steadman, 1989; Winters and Rich, 1998). In treatment-seeking samples, between 10% and 44% of those identified with gambling disorder reported that one or more of their parents had a gambling problem (Daghestani et al., 1996; Gambino et al., 1993; Lesieur and Blume, 1990; Lesieur and Heineman, 1988; Lesieur et al., 1986). Although cross-sectional studies suggest gambling disorder has a heritable component, these types of studies are unable to distinguish the extent to which gambling among family members results from genetic or environmental influences.

Twin studies can tease out the role between shared environment and genetics. In the earliest such study of gambling disorder, Winters and Rich (1998) reported greater similarity of gambling among 42 monozygotic twin pairs compared with 50 dizygotic twin pairs, but the effect was noted only among men and only among those who played games with high potential payoffs, such as casino cards, gambling machines, pull tabs, and lottery. The association was not significant for lower payoff games such as informal card betting, bingo, and games of personal skill or among women. Similar to the results of studies of alcoholism (McGue et al., 1992), the genetic risk for gambling appeared stronger in men than in women.

In a study of 6,718 men participating in the Vietnam Era Twin Registry, Eisen et al. (1998) examined vulnerability from inherited factors, shared environmental experiences, and non-shared environmental experiences. Shared environmental experiences include exposure to parental gambling and having the same childhood friends—experiences assumed to contribute equally to risk in monozygotic and dizygotic twins. Unique environmental influences involve experiences outside, or not shared within, the family. Familial factors (inheritance and/or shared childhood experiences) explained 62% of the variance in development of gambling disorder. A follow-up study of this same sample (Slutske et al., 2000) revealed a linear relationship between severity of alcohol and gambling disorders: The percentages of participants with no, mild, moderate, and severe alcohol dependence who were also diagnosed with gambling disorder were 0.7%, 0.8%, 2.5%, and 4.5%, respectively. Slutske and colleagues (2000) also estimated that 64%–75% of the co-occurrence of gambling and alcohol use disorders related to genes that influenced both disorders simultaneously, whereas shared family environmental experiences did not contribute to the development of these disorders. Unique environmental experiences influenced both gambling and alcohol use disorders, but these non-shared environmental experiences were responsible for considerably less of the overlap between disorders than the genetic factors. In a related study, Slutske et al. (2001) also found that the comorbidity between gambling and antisocial personality disorder was explained primarily by genetic factors rather than environmental ones. Impulsive behavior patterns characterize antisocial personality disorder, perhaps in part explaining the link between impulsivity, neurocognitive function, and gambling and substance use disorders described previously.

Studies of the molecular genetics of gambling disorder focus primarily on the involvement of the brain's reward system in addictions, with dopamine genes a primary target of study. The dopamine 2 receptor gene (DRD2) is implicated in the reward deficiency syndrome (Blum et al., 1995; Comings and Blum, 2000). Early studies found an association between gambling disorder and a polymorphism of the T allele of the DRD2 gene (Comings et al., 1996b, 1997). A polymorphism in the DRD1 gene may also play a role in the neurobiology of gambling and alcohol disorders (Comings et al., 1997; da Silva Lobo et al., 2007). A study of a Korean sample, however, found no association between dopamine receptor genes and gambling disorder (Lim et al., 2012), but that study was quite small. Similarly, in a Canadian sample, Lobo et al. (2010) did not find an association between any single polymorphism investigated on DRD1 and DRD3 receptor genes and gambling, but they observed trends with respect to a TaqIA/rs1800497 polymorphism and the DRD2 gene. A polymorphism in the DRD4 gene has been associated with impulsivity (Benjamin et al., 1996; Ebstein et al., 1996; Strobel et al., 1999) and linked with gambling disorder as well (Comings et al., 1999), although this effect was noted only in females in one sample (Perez de Castro et al., 1997).

In contrast, a variant in the promoter region of the serotonin transporter gene (5-HTTLPR) contributed to the risk of gambling disorder in men (Comings et al., 1997), and severe forms of gambling disorder in men relate to a polymorphism allele in the promoter region of the monoamine oxidase A (MAO-A) gene (Ibanez et al., 2000; Perez de Castro et al., 2002). Wilson et al. (2013) investigated polymorphisms of serotonin transporter genes in 140 sibling pairs discordant for gambling disorder. They found a significant association between a genotype of the serotonin receptor 2A T102C and gambling disorder, consistent with reports for nicotine and alcohol dependence (Jakubczyk et al., 2012; White et al., 2011).

Comings et al. (1996a) found mutations in the serotonin tryptophan 2,3-dioxygenese (TDO2) gene in individuals with gambling disorder. Subsequently, Comings et al. (2001) used a genetic technique to evaluate the additive effects of multiple genes in 139 individuals with gambling disorder and 139 controls. Two serotonin genes related to gambling disorder—the *TPH* and *TDO2* genes. The *TPH* gene is associated with suicidality and alcoholism (Nielsen et al., 1998), and in this study, a greater association of the *TPH* gene occurred among the gamblers with a history of substance abuse than gamblers without such a history. In contrast, the *TDO2* gene was present primarily in gamblers with no history of substance abuse, consistent with a prior study showing this gene was unrelated to alcoholism (Comings et al., 1996a). In this sample (Comings et al., 2001), dopamine genes also contributed to the risk of gambling disorder, although the variance accounted for was small.

Lind et al. (2013) performed a genome-wide association study of gambling disorder in 1,312 Australian twins. Although no single-nucleotide polymorphisms (SNPs) reached genome-wide significance, six were implicated in gambling disorder. Two SNPs were on chromosome 9, and one was near chromosome 12; several addiction-related pathways were enriched for SNPs associated with gambling disorder as well. Thus, the available data on the molecular genetics of gambling disorder are consistent with the comorbidity of gambling and substance use disorders and the neurobiology of impulsivity. Further identification of genes and biological pathways may help characterize biological mechanisms underlying gambling disorder and possibly response to its treatment.

TREATMENTS

As in substance use disorders, relatively few persons with gambling disorder present for treatment. In epidemiological samples, less than 10% of individuals with gambling disorder have ever sought treatment for it (Slutske, 2006). Those who seek services tend to have more severe symptoms or external pressures, such as legal, employment, or family difficulties, prompting treatment entry. For those who do present for services, a number of treatments appear effective. Most are based on treatments for substance use disorders, such as 12-step therapies and cognitive–behavioral, cognitive, and brief motivational interventions. In addition, several medications have been tested for treating gambling disorder, although none are approved for this indication.

Gamblers Anonymous

Alcoholics Anonymous is the most widely accessed intervention for substance use disorders in the United States, and its counterpart for gambling disorder is Gamblers Anonymous (GA). Although GA exists throughout the United States and in many other countries throughout the world, there are little data related to its effectiveness. Among the earliest reports is an observation study from Scotland. Stewart and Brown (1988) followed 232 gamblers for 1 year who attended a GA meeting. They found that only 8% remained engaged in the organization and maintained gambling abstinence for 1 year. GA may engender more positive effects when it is combined with professionally delivered therapy. In a longitudinal observation of 342 individuals receiving professional gambling therapy (Petry, 2003), 36% of patients who attended professional care alone achieved and maintained gambling abstinence compared with 48% of those who also attended GA. Although suggestive of benefits, selection biases may have impacted outcomes because those who also attended GA may have been more motivated to stop gambling. No randomized trials of the efficacy of GA exist.

AA may have many GA's in recovery

Cognitive–Behavioral Therapy

Randomized studies of other interventions have been conducted and do demonstrate benefits. Petry (2005) developed an eight-session cognitive–behavioral therapy (CBT) and evaluated its efficacy in a randomized clinical trial of 235 individuals with gambling disorder. The three treatments were referral to GA, referral to GA plus CBT presented in the context of a self-directed workbook, or referral to GA plus CBT delivered by a trained counselor in weekly individual sessions. The CBT was identical in the two latter conditions, and Petry describes it in full. The CBT consists of eight topics: identification of triggers, functional analysis of gambling, engaging in alternative activities, self-management of triggers, coping with urges to gamble, gambling refusal skills, dispelling cognitive distortions, and relapse prevention.

Participants assigned to the professionally delivered CBT condition evidenced the greatest reductions in gambling. Not only did gambling decrease more substantially but also these participants experienced greater reductions in psychiatric symptoms, and improvements were maintained throughout the 12-month follow-up period. This study included important design features to validate these results. The vast majority of participants in all three of the conditions completed follow-up evaluations throughout a 12-month post-treatment period, and all participants were included in the analyses using an intent-to-treat approach. In addition, friends or relatives who were aware of the participant's gambling provided independent evaluations of the participant's gambling behavior as an independent corroboration of self-reports. Participants in all three conditions reported equal rates of participation in GA, suggesting that the benefits in this professionally delivered CBT condition occurred independently of GA attendance.

Participants in the CBT workbook condition, however, did not reduce gambling any more than those assigned to GA alone. Differential rates of participation in CBT explained the discrepancies in response to it. Only 37% of those in the CBT workbook condition completed at least six of the eight chapters, but 61% assigned to professionally delivered CBT attended at least six sessions. The number of CBT exercises completed related to reductions in gambling, and development of new coping skills from pre- to post-treatment mediated the effects of the intervention on gambling outcomes (Petry et al., 2008), indicating that skills taught in the CBT had the intended effects. Morasco et al. (2006) provide details of internal and external precipitants of gambling and patients' responses to them.

Other studies have also noted reductions in gambling with CBT, although most other study designs involved wait-list control conditions, which limit conclusions that can be drawn from them because of expectancy effects as well as inability to ascertain long-term post-treatment benefits. In Sweden, Carlbring and Smit (2008) randomized 66 gamblers to an Internet-delivered CBT, which involved some therapist contact via e-mail and phone calls, or a wait-list control condition. The Internet CBT condition reduced gambling to a greater extent than the control condition during the study period. However, because participants assigned to the wait-list condition received the intervention after 8 weeks, this study could not ascertain long-term benefits. In a second study, Carlbring et al. (2012) followed 316 gamblers for 36 months after they initiated online CBT gambling treatment. Reductions in gambling occurred throughout the study period, but whether these effects were related to the intervention or reflective of participant characteristics could not be determined because no control condition was included. Furthermore, engagement in the CBT was relatively low, with only 44% of enrolled participants completing the online sessions. Thus, although appropriate for some gamblers, self-directed CBT, online or via workbooks, is unlikely to engage patients to the same extent as therapists. Nevertheless, CBT, especially when delivered by therapists, can be effective in reducing gambling.

Cognitive Therapy

Most studies of CBT included one or more sessions related to dispelling irrational cognitions related to gambling, such as overestimating the odds of winning or feeling able to predict when a win is due. Some studies applying an entirely cognitive approach address these illusions throughout the course of treatment. For example, Ladouceur et al. (2001) randomized 59 gamblers to cognitive therapy or a wait-list control condition. The cognitive therapy included up to 20 sessions, or until the patient stopped gambling. In total, 59% of those receiving cognitive therapy completed treatment and reduced gambling. In a subsequent study, Ladouceur et al. (2003) applied this same therapy in a group context. Seventy-one gamblers were randomly assigned to group cognitive therapy or a wait-list control condition. Again, reductions in gambling were more pronounced in those in the cognitive therapy condition than in those in the wait-list condition. However, expectancy effects may have impacted outcomes, and wait-list control designs preclude examination of long-term efficacy.

Brief and Motivational Interventions

In contrast to the fairly intensive cognitive therapy approach, other studies have examined the efficacy of brief interventions for gambling. Motivational interviewing (MI) and motivational enhancement therapy (MET), were designed as minimal interventions for substance use disorders. MI refers to an interviewing style in which the therapist meets the patients where they are and attempts to point out discrepancies in their desire to continue versus reduce their problem behavior, with the goal of increasing their motivation to reduce the problem behavior. MET usually consists of two to four sessions, based on these techniques.

These MI and MET approaches appear to reduce gambling. Hodgins et al. (2001) randomly assigned 102 gamblers to one of three conditions: a wait-list control, a workbook containing CBT exercises, or a single MI telephone session with the CBT workbook. The CBT workbook alone did not lead to greater reductions in gambling than the wait-list condition, but it did when combined with MI. Follow-up assessments, restricted to patients assigned to the non-wait-list conditions, found that some benefits of MI were maintained after the treatment period ended. In a larger follow-up study, Hodgins et al. (2009) randomized 314 gamblers to a 6-week wait-list control condition, a workbook-only control condition, or one of two brief interventions. One brief intervention involved a single session using MI along with a mailed CBT workbook. The second applied the same approach but added six booster telephone calls over a 9-month period. Both brief interventions resulted in less gambling than the control conditions at a 6-week evaluation. However, the participants assigned to the CBT workbook-only condition were as likely as those assigned to MI to decrease gambling throughout the remainder of the year. The booster calls did not result in any added benefits. Data from these studies suggest that brief treatments can be effective, but more treatment does not necessarily confer greater benefits.

Other studies applied MI and MET during in-person sessions, as opposed to over the phone. Grant et al. (2009) randomized 68 gamblers to receive MI followed by CBT or referral to GA and found benefits of the MI–CBT approach. Oei et al. (2010) randomized 102 gamblers to MI + CBT delivered in individual sessions, MI + CBT delivered in group sessions, or a 6-week wait-list control condition. Significant improvements were noted in both MI + CBT conditions compared to the control condition post-treatment, and the format of the therapy did not impact outcomes.

The previous studies all evaluated MI or MET in conjunction with CBT. Others have found benefits of MI on its own. Petry et al. (2009) randomized 117 problem gambling college students to an assessment-only control condition, 10 minutes of brief advice, one 50-minute session of MI, or one session of MI plus three sessions of CBT. All treatments were provided on an individual basis, and the brief advice involved provision of personal feedback and specific suggestions for reducing gambling. Compared to the control condition, students who received any of the active treatments reduced gambling, but only the MI condition maintained significant reductions in gambling relative to the control condition at a 9-month follow-up evaluation.

In a study with a similar design, Petry et al. (2008) screened patients at low-income medical clinics and substance abuse treatment clinics for gambling problems. A total of 180 patients identified with gambling problems were randomized to the four treatments outlined previously. Outcomes in the three active conditions again did not differ significantly, but in this study, those assigned to the brief advice condition experienced the greatest reductions in gambling. Results across studies suggest that brief interventions can be efficacious in reducing gambling, although the content and duration of the intervention with the most pronounced effects may vary across populations. In particular, students may be more likely to benefit from nondirective motivational approaches, whereas adult indigent populations may respond best to very targeted, direct, and brief approaches.

Importantly, neither of these studies included "treatment-seeking" gamblers in the traditional sense. Instead, they applied these approaches to individuals who screened positive for gambling problems and probably would be very unlikely to seek services on their own.

In Canada, Cunningham et al. (2012) randomized 209 gamblers to a wait-list control condition or one of two feedback conditions. The first integrated feedback about one's gambling in relation to population norms; the second also gave feedback about one's gambling, but it did not involve comparisons to the general population. In this study, the full feedback and control conditions did not differ with respect to gambling outcomes, but the partial feedback condition resulted in less gambling. Together, these data, similarly to those reported by Petry et al. (2008, 2009), suggest that a single session may be sufficient to reduce gambling in some gamblers, but the content and duration of efficacious brief interventions require further study, along with a better understanding of persons most likely to benefit from minimal intervention approaches.

Pharmacotherapies

The U.S. Food and Drug Administration has not approved any medication for the treatment of gambling disorder. However, several pharmacotherapies have undergone investigation for treating this disorder. Three broad categories of pharmacotherapies have been tested: opioid antagonists, antidepressants, and mood stabilizers. Many initial studies of these medications involved open-label drug administration without a placebo control. These designs led to an overinflation of effects (Pallesen et al., 2007). Here, only medication trials that included a placebo control condition are reviewed.

Naltrexone and nalmefene are opioid antagonists, which are drugs that block the effects of endogenous endorphins on the central opiate receptors. Opioid antagonists can also have effects related to inhibiting dopamine release in the nucleus accumbens, a region of the brain involved with reward. Opioid antagonists are typically used to treat substance use disorders, and several studies have evaluated their efficacy for reducing gambling as well. For example, Grant et al. (2006) conducted a 16-week randomized, double-blind, placebo-controlled trial of nalmefene. In total, 207 patients with gambling disorder were randomized to placebo or nalmefene at one of three doses: 25, 50, or 100 mg/day. Patients treated with the two lower doses of nalmefene evidenced greater reductions in gambling compared to those randomized to the placebo condition. However, significant adverse medication effects were noted, especially among those receiving higher doses. In a subsequent study, Grant et al. (2010) randomized 233 patients with gambling disorder to placebo or 20 or 40 mg per day doses of nalmefene. Using an intent-to-treat approach, nalmefene failed to improve outcomes on any measure. Post hoc analyses of only participants who received a full titration of the medication and remained in treatment for at least 1 week demonstrated that the higher dose resulted in some reductions in gambling compared to those for placebo-treated participants. These findings suggest that dosing may be important but that opioid antagonists are not well tolerated, especially at higher doses.

Medications used in the treatment of depression have also been applied to treat gambling disorder, but these have generally resulted in mixed or modest effects. For example, Kim et al. (2002) conducted a double-blind study comparing paroxetine to placebo in 45 patients, and they found that paroxetine led to greater reductions in gambling urges compared to placebo. Another trial compared fluvoxamine to placebo in 32 patients but showed no benefit of the medication (Blanco et al., 2002). Saiz-Ruiz et al. (2005) evaluated sertraline and placebo in 60 patients with gambling disorder and found no benefit of this antidepressant medication. Thus, there is limited evidence of efficacy for antidepressants in treating gambling disorder.

Mood stabilizers have been evaluated in treating comorbid gambling and bipolar disorder. Hollander et al. (2005) conducted a double-blind, placebo-controlled study of lithium carbonate among 40 individuals with co-occurring gambling and bipolar spectrum disorders. They found that lithium reduced gambling symptoms to a greater extent than placebo. These data suggest potential for mood stabilizers in the treatment of gambling in this dual-diagnosis population. Nevertheless, additional research is needed to better understand the short- and long-term efficacy of pharmacotherapies in the treatment of gambling disorder. Furthermore, as noted by Pallesen et al. (2007), the effect sizes of pharmacotherapies appear to be smaller than those associated with psychotherapies. The lower effect sizes may relate to the inclusion of better control conditions in double-blind randomized pharmacotherapy studies relative to many psychotherapy studies. In addition, the patients choosing to participate in different types of studies may differ in gambling severity, rendering them more or less likely to respond favorably to treatments. As the field moves forward, greater consensus must be achieved in terms of classifying patients with gambling disorder who participate in research studies and how gambling and related problems are assessed at the time of study initiation and throughout the course of treatment.

FUTURE DIRECTIONS

Moving gambling disorders to the substance use and related addictive disorders section of the DSM-5 holds potential to open opportunities for better understanding, preventing, and treating this behavioral addiction. With gambling aligned with substance use disorders, clinicians treating patients with substance use disorder may be more likely to screen for, and treat when indicated, gambling problems. As noted previously, some brief screens exist to rapidly identify individuals who may benefit from further assessment. Further development and assessment of the psychometric properties of brief instruments for gambling disorders could increase the proportion of individuals who are screened for, and offered, gambling treatment.

As with substance use disorders, however, screening and identification alone do not necessarily result in accessing treatment. Far more individuals with addictive disorders do not receive services than those who do. Longitudinal studies need to assess the natural course of gambling disorder and how it waxes and wanes over time—with and without treatment. Identification of predictors of those who recover naturally, without intervention, can help to direct intervention efforts to those most in need of them. For those who are unlikely to cease gambling on their own, development and refinement of interventions acceptable to individuals who screen positive for gambling problems are necessary.

Because many of the existing interventions for gambling disorder are based on those developed for substance use disorders, integrating gambling-specific interventions theoretically should be relatively straightforward for providers familiar with treating substance use disorders. Nevertheless, there are some important distinguishing features between the presentation of gambling and substance use disorders. For example, substance abuse treatment providers are largely unfamiliar with gambling and the extent of its consequences. The financial repercussions of gambling disorder are often paramount, and few substance abuse providers are familiar with assisting patients with financial concerns. In addition, substance abuse providers are skilled at recognizing overt effects of substance use and intoxication, many of which are physiologically apparent. In contrast, there are no overt symptoms of gambling and no objective index on which to gauge one's progress in terms of reducing gambling. Therefore, special training in monitoring gambling-specific symptoms and progress may be necessary.

Although evidence-based treatments such as CBT, MI, and MET exist for substance use disorders, few community-based treatment providers are experienced in providing these treatments. Introducing gambling interventions into the context of substance abuse treatment services holds potential to train providers in these techniques. Providers may be more open to applying new interventions toward treating gambling than they are to substance use disorders. If clinicians observe these approaches working well in terms of decreasing gambling, they may then be inclined to use these interventions in the treatment of substance use disorders as well.

Although CBT, MI, and MET show promise in treating gambling disorder, more research must establish their efficacy. No published studies have included attention control conditions that equate expectancy effects. Few interventions have been studied in more than one trial or across multiple investigators. Rarely have studies used intent-to-treat analyses, and many gambling treatment studies do not reach scientifically acceptable standards in terms of quality.

In addition, because many persons successfully reduce gambling at least in the short term upon initiating treatment, studies need to evaluate long-term effects of interventions that demonstrate initial efficacy during the treatment period. Few gambling treatment studies have applied sophisticated data analytic strategies to evaluate changes in gambling and other symptoms over time, taking into account within and across group and person variances for missing data, which are inevitable in clinical trials.

Relatedly, no generally accepted standard exists for evaluating gambling outcomes. Across studies, outcomes include self-reports of frequencies and/or quantities of self-reports of gambling behavior, urges or desires to gamble, and DSM symptom counts. Pharmacological trials generally rely on different scales and outcome measures than those used in psychotherapy trials. Very few studies include independent validators of gambling. Researchers need to achieve a consensus about measures that best assess gambling outcomes.

Finally, uncovering robust predictors of the development of gambling problems will help guide prevention and early intervention efforts. To date, little research has addressed methods to prevent gambling problems, and no approaches have demonstrated promise in preventing gambling problems. Given the increasing acceptance and legalization of gambling opportunities in the United States and countries throughout the world, and the increasing access to Internet gaming, prevention of gambling disorder is of upmost concern.

If neurobiological or genetic markers of gambling disorder are discovered, targeted prevention or intervention efforts may also be possible. For example, pharmacotherapies that correct neurocognitive deficits may be best directed toward gamblers with physiological deficiencies. Individuals with gambling disorder who do not evidence physiological abnormalities, in contrast, may benefit from psychotherapies. A better understanding of the neurophysiology of gambling disorder may also elucidate how interventions—be they pharmacological or psychological—exert their beneficial effects. If interventions reverse impulsive decision-making, such approaches may also be useful in treating other addictive disorders with similar underlying neurocognitive features. Interventions that reverse cognitive or functional deficits in decision-making processes may also be applicable in the context of preventing gambling and possibly other behavioral addictions as well.

Finally, given the high rates of comorbidities and similarities across behavioral addictions, discoveries from gambling research may facilitate efforts in other addictions. If a common genetic or neurophysiological process underlies behavioral addictions, then effective prevention and intervention efforts may inform multiple disorders. Because research is only emerging in many of these newer conditions, lessons learned can be applied in other contexts to more rapidly advance our understanding of the etiology, treatment, and prevention of behavioral addictions.

REFERENCES

Abbott, M.W., Volberg, R.A., 2000. Taking the pulse on gambling and problem gambling in New Zealand: A report on phase one of the 1999 National Prevalence Survey. Wellington, New Zealand: Department of Internal Affairs.

American Psychiatric Association, 2013. *Diagnostic and statistical manual of mental disorders* (5th ed.). Washington, DC: American Psychiatric Association.

Asensio, S., Romero, M.J., Palau, C., Sanchez, A., Senabre, I., Morales, J.L., et al., 2010. Altered neural response of the appetitive emotional system in cocaine addiction: An fMRI study. Addict Biol. 15, 504–516.

Balodis, I.M., Kober, H., Worhunsky, P.D., Stevens, M.C., Pearlson, G.D., Potenza, M.N., 2012. Diminished frontostriatal activity during processing of monetary rewards and losses in pathological gambling. Biol Psychiatry. 71, 749–757.

Benjamin, J., Li, L., Patterson, C., Greenberg, B.D., Murphy, D.L., Hamer, D.H., 1996. Population and familial association between the D4 dopamine receptor gene and measures of Novelty Seeking. Nat Genet. 12, 81–84.

Blanco, C., Petkova, E., Ibanez, A., Saiz-Ruiz, J., 2002. A pilot placebo-controlled study of fluvoxamine for pathological gambling. Ann Clin Psychiatry. 14, 9–15.

Blum, K., Sheridan, P.J., Wood, R.C., Braverman, E.R., Chen, T.J., Comings, D.E., 1995. Dopamine D2 receptor gene variants: Association and linkage studies in impulsive–addictive–compulsive behaviour. Pharmacogenetics. 5, 121–141.

Bondolfi, G., Osiek, C., Ferrero, F., 2000. Prevalence estimates of pathological gambling in Switzerland. Acta Psychiatr Scand. 101, 473–475.

Carlbring, P., Smit, F., 2008. Randomized trial of Internet-delivered self-help with telephone support for pathological gamblers. J Consult Clin Psychol. 76, 1090–1094.

Carlbring, P., Degerman, N., Jonsson, J., Andersson, G., 2012. Internet-based treatment of pathological gambling with a three-year follow-up. Cogn Behav Ther. 41, 321–334.

Chassin, L., Fora, D.B., King, K.M., 2004. Trajectories of alcohol and drug use and dependence from adolescence to adulthood: The effects of familial alcoholism and personality. J Abnorm Psychol. 113, 483–498.

Comings, D.E., Gade, R., Muhleman, D., Chiu, C., Wu, S., To, M., et al., 1996a. Exon and intron variants in the human tryptophan 2,3-dioxygenase gene: Potential association with Tourette syndrome, substance abuse and other disorders. Pharmacogenetics. 6, 307–318.

Comings, D.E., Rosenthal, R.J., Lesieur, H.R., Rugle, L.J., Muhleman, D., Chiu, C., et al., 1996b. A study of the dopamine D2 receptor gene in pathological gambling. Pharmacogenetics. 6, 223–234.

Comings, D.E., Gade, R., Wu, S., Chiu, C., Dietz, G., Muhleman, D., et al., 1997. Studies of the potential role of the dopamine D1 receptor gene in addictive behaviors. Mol Psychiatry. 2, 44–56.

Comings, D.E., Gonzalez, N., Wu, S., Gade, R., Muhleman, D., Saucier, G., et al., 1999. Studies of the 48 bp repeat polymorphism of the DRD4 gene in impulsive, compulsive, addictive behaviors: Tourette syndrome, ADHD, pathological gambling, and substance abuse. Am J Med Genet. 88, 358–368.

Comings, D.E., Blum, K., 2000. Reward deficiency syndrome: Genetic aspects of behavioral disorders. Prog Brain Res. 126, 325–341.

Comings, D.E., Gade-Andavolu, R., Gonzalez, N., Wu, S., Muhleman, D., Chen, C., et al., 2001. The additive effect of neurotransmitter genes in pathological gambling. Clin Genet. 60, 107–116.

Cunningham, J.A., Hodgins, D.C., Toneatto, T., Murphy, M., 2012. A randomized controlled trial of a personalized feedback intervention for problem gamblers. PLoS ONE. 7, e31586.

Currie, S.R., Hodgins, D.C., Casey, D.M., 2013. Validity of the Problem Gambling Severity Index interpretive categories. J Gambl Stud. 29, 311–327.

da Silva Lobo, D.S., Vallada, H.P., Knight, J., Martins, S.S., Tavares, H., Gentil, V., et al., 2007. Dopamine genes and pathological gambling in discordant sib-pairs. J Gambl Stud. 23, 421–433.

Daghestani, A.N., Elenz, E., Crayton, J.W., 1996. Pathological gambling in hospitalized substance abusing veterans. J Clin Psychiatry. 57, 360–363.

Delfabbro, P., King, D., Lambos, C., Puglies, S., 2009. Is video-game playing a risk factor for pathological gambling in Australian adolescents? J Gambl Stud. 25, 391–405.

Ebstein, R.P., Novick, O., Umansky, R., Priel, B., Osher, Y., Blaine, D., et al., 1996. Dopamine D4 receptor (D4DR) exon III polymorphism associated with the human personality trait of Novelty Seeking. Nat Genet. 12, 78–80.

Eisen, S.A., Lin, N., Lyons, M.J., Scherrer, J.F., Griffith, K., True, W.R., et al., 1998. Familial influences on gambling behavior: An analysis of 3359 twin pairs. Addiction. 93, 1375–1384.

el-Guebaly, N., Patten, S.B., Currie, S., Williams, J.V., Beck, C.A., Maxwell, C.J., et al., 2006. Epidemiological associations between gambling behavior, substance use & mood and anxiety disorders. J Gambl Stud. 22, 275–287.

Evenden, J., 1999. Impulsivity: A discussion of clinical and experimental findings. J Psychopharmacol. 13, 180–192.

Ferris, J., Wynne, H., 2001. The Canadian problem gambling index. Ottawa, ON: Canadian Centre on Substance Abuse.

Gambino, B., Fitzgerald, R., Shaffer, H., Benner, J., Courtnage, P., 1993. Perceived family history of problem gambling and scores on SOGS. J Gambl Stud. 9, 169–184.

Gerstein, D., Murphy, S., Toce, M., Hoffmann, J., Palmer, A., Johnson, R., et al., 1999. Gambling Impact and Behavior Study: A Report to the National Gambling Impact Study Commission. Chicago: National Opinion Research Center.

Gotestam, K.G., Johansson, A., 2003. Characteristics of gambling and problematic gambling in the Norwegian context: A DSM-IV-based telephone interview study. Addict Behav. 28, 189–197.

Grant, B.F., Dawson, D.A., Stinson, F.S., Chou, P.S., Kay, W., Pickering, R., 2003. The Alcohol Use Disorder and Associated Disabilities Interview Schedule-IV (AUDADIS-IV): Reliability of alcohol consumption, tobacco use, family history of depression and psychiatric diagnostic modules in a general population sample. Drug Alcohol Depend. 71, 7–16.

Grant, J.E., Potenza, M.N., Hollander, E., Cunningham-Williams, R., Nurminen, T., Smits, G., et al., 2006. Multicenter investigation of the opioid antagonist nalmefene in the treatment of pathological gambling. Am J Psychiatry. 163, 303–312.

Grant, J.E., Donahue, C.B., Odlaug, B.L., Kim, S.W., Miller, M.J., Petry, N.M., 2009. Imaginal desensitisation plus motivational interviewing for pathological gambling: Randomised controlled trial. Br J Psychiatry. 195, 266–267.

Grant, J.E., Odlaug, B.L., Potenza, M.N., Hollander, E., Kim, S.W., 2010. Nalmefene in the treatment of pathological gambling: Multicentre, double-blind, placebo-controlled study. Br J Psychiatry. 197, 330–331.

Guo, J., Hawkins, J.D., Hill, K.G., Abbott, R.D., 2001. Childhood and adolescent predictors of alcohol abuse and dependence in young adulthood. J Stud Alcohol. 62, 754–762.

Hawkins, J.D., Catalano, R.F., Miller, J.Y., 1992. Risk and protective factors for alcohol and other drug problems in adolescence and early adulthood: Implications for substance abuse prevention. Psychol Bull. 112, 64–105.

Hill, K.G., White, H.R., Chung, I.J., Hawkins, J.D., Catalano, R.F., 2000. Early adult outcomes of adolescent binge drinking: Person- and variable-centered analyses of binge drinking trajectories. Alcohol Clin Exp Res. 24, 892–901.

Hodgins, D.C., 2004. Using the NORC DSM Screen for Gambling Problems as an outcome measure for pathological gambling: Psychometric evaluation. Addict Behav. 29, 1685–1690.

Hodgins, D.C., Currie, S.R., el-Guebaly, N., 2001. Motivational enhancement and self-help treatments for problem gambling. J Consult Clin Psychol. 69, 50–57.

Hodgins, D.C., Currie, S.R., Currie, G., Fick, G.H., 2009. Randomized trial of brief motivational treatments for pathological gamblers: More is not necessarily better. J Consult Clin Psychol. 77, 950–960.

Hollander, E., Pallanti, S., Allen, A., Sood, E., Baldini Rossi, N., 2005. Does sustained-release lithium reduce impulsive gambling and affective instability versus placebo in pathological gamblers with bipolar spectrum disorders? Am J Psychiatry. 162, 137–145.

Hommer, D.W., Bjork, J.M., Gilman, J.M., 2011. Imaging brain response to reward in addictive disorders. Ann N Y Acad Sci. 1216, 50–61.

Ibanez, A., Perez de Castro, I., Fernandez-Piqueras, J., Blanco, C., Saiz-Ruiz, J., 2000. Pathological gambling and DNA polymorphic markers at MAO-A and MAO-B genes. Mol Psychiatry. 5, 105–109.

Jia, Z., Worhunsky, P.D., Carroll, K.M., Rounsaville, B.J., Stevens, M.C., Pearlson, G.D., Potenza, M.N., 2011. An initial study of neural responses to monetary incentives as related to treatment outcome in cocaine dependence. Biol Psychiatry. 70(6), 553–560.

Jakubczyk, A., Wrzosek, M., Lukaszkiewicz, J., Sadowska-Mazuryk, J., Matsumoto, H., Sliwerska, E., et al., 2012. The CC genotype in HTR2A T102C polymorphism is associated with behavioral impulsivity in alcohol-dependent patients. J Psychiatr Res. 46, 44–49.

Joutsa, J., Saunavaara, J., Parkkola, R., Niemela, S., Kaasinen, V., 2011. Extensive abnormality of brain white matter integrity in pathological gambling. Psychiatry Res. 194, 340–346.

Kandel, D.B., Kessler, R.C., Margulies, R.Z., 1978. Antecedents of adolescent initiation into stages of drug use: A developmental analysis. J Youth Adolesc. 7, 13–40.

Kessler, R.C., Hwang, I., LaBrie, R., Petukhova, M., Sampson, N.A., Winters, K.C., et al., 2008. DSM-IV pathological gambling in the National Comorbidity Survey Replication. Psychol Med. 38, 1351–1360.

Kim, S.W., Grant, J.E., Adson, D.E., Shin, Y.C., Zaninelli, R., 2002. A double-blind placebo-controlled study of the efficacy and safety of paroxetine in the treatment of pathological gambling. J Clin Psychiatry. 63, 501–507.

Ladouceur, R., Sylvain, C., Boutin, C., Lachance, S., Doucet, C., Leblond, J., et al., 2001. Cognitive treatment of pathological gambling. J Nerv Ment Dis. 189, 774–780.

Ladouceur, R., Sylvain, C., Boutin, C., Lachance, S., Doucet, C., Leblond, J., 2003. Group therapy for pathological gamblers: A cognitive approach. Behav Res Ther. 41, 587–596.

Lee, Y.S., Han, D.H., Kim, S.M., Renshaw, P.F., 2013. Substance abuse precedes Internet addiction. Addict Behav. 38, 2022–2025.

Lesieur, H.R., Blume, S.B., Zoppa, R.M., 1986. Alcoholism, drug abuse, and gambling. Alcohol Clin Exp Res. 10, 33–38.

Lesieur, H.R., Blume, S.B., 1987. The South Oaks Gambling Screen (SOGS): A new instrument for the identification of pathological gamblers. Am J Psychiatry. 144, 1184–1188.

Lesieur, H.R., Heineman, M., 1988. Pathological gambling among youthful multiple substance abusers in a therapeutic community. Br J Addict. 83, 765–771.

Lesieur, H.R., Blume, S.B., 1990. Characteristics of pathological gamblers identified among patients on a psychiatric admissions service. Hosp Community Psychiatry. 41, 1009–1012.

Lim, S., Ha, J., Choi, S.W., Kang, S.G., Shin, Y.C., 2012. Association study on pathological gambling and polymorphisms of dopamine D1, D2, D3, and D4 receptor genes in a Korean population. J Gambl Stud. 28, 481–491.

Lind, P.A., Zhu, G., Montgomery, G.W., Madden, P.A., Heath, A.C., Martin, N.G., et al., 2013. Genome-wide association study of a quantitative disordered gambling trait. Addict Biol. 18, 511–522.

Lobo, D.S., Souza, R.P., Tong, R.P., Casey, D.M., Hodgins, D.C., Smith, G.J., et al., 2010. Association of functional variants in the dopamine D2-like receptors with risk for gambling behaviour in healthy Caucasian subjects. Biol Psychol. 85, 33–37.

Lorains, F.K., Cowlishaw, S., Thomas, S.A., 2011. Prevalence of comorbid disorders in problem and pathological gambling: Systematic review and meta-analysis of population surveys. Addiction. 106, 490–498.

Lund, I., Nordlund, S., 2003. Gambling and problem gambling in Norway. SIRUS Report No. 2. Oslo: Norwegian Institute for Alcohol and Drug Research.

Martinez, D., Narendran, R., Foltin, R.W., Slifstein, M., Hwang, D.R., Broft, A., et al., 2007. Amphetamine-induced dopamine release: Markedly blunted in cocaine dependence and predictive of the choice to self-administer cocaine. Am J Psychiatry. 164, 622–629.

McGue, M., Pickens, R.W., Svikis, D.S., 1992. Sex and age effects on the inheritance of alcohol problems: A twin study. J Abnorm Psychol. 101, 3–17.

McGue, M., Slutske, W., Taylor, J., Iacono, W.G., 1997. Personality and substance use disorders: I. Effects of gender and alcoholism subtype. Alcohol Clin Exp Res. 21, 513–520.

Miedl, S.F., Fehr, T., Meyer, G., Herrmann, M., 2010. Neurobiological correlates of problem gambling in a quasi-realistic blackjack scenario as revealed by fMRI. Psychiatry Res. 181, 165–173.

Miedl, S.F., Peters, J., Buchel, C., 2012. Altered neural reward representations in pathological gamblers revealed by delay and probability discounting. Arch Gen Psychiatry. 69, 177–186.

Ministry of Community Development, 2005. Report of survey on participation in gambling activities among Singapore residents, 2005. Singapore: National Council on Problem Gambling.

Morasco, B.J., Pietrzak, R.H., Blanco, C., Grant, B.F., Hasin, D., Petry, N.M., 2006. Health problems and medical utilization associated with gambling disorders: Results from the National Epidemiologic Survey on Alcohol and Related Conditions. Psychosom Med. 68, 976–984.

Nielsen, D.A., Virkkunen, M., Lappalainen, J., Eggert, M., Brown, G.L., Long, J.C., et al., 1998. A tryptophan hydroxylase gene marker for suicidality and alcoholism. Arch Gen Psychiatry. 55, 593–602.

Oei, T.P., Raylu, N., Casey, L.M., 2010. Effectiveness of group and individual formats of a combined motivational interviewing and cognitive behavioral treatment program for problem gambling: A randomized controlled trial. Behav Cogn Psychother. 38, 233–238.

Orford, J., Sproston, K., Erens, B., 2003. SOGS and DSM-IV in the British Gambling Prevalence Survey: Reliability and factor structure. International Gambling Studies. 3, 53–65.

Orford, J., Wardle, H., Griffiths, M., Sproston, K., Erens, B., 2010. PGSI and DSM-IV in the 2007 British Gambling Prevalence Survey: Reliability, item response, factor structure and inter-scale agreement. International Gambling Studies. 10, 31–44.

Pagani, L.S., Derevensky, J.L., Japel, C., 2009. Predicting gambling behavior in sixth grade from kindergarten impulsivity: A tale of developmental continuity. Arch Pediatr Adolesc Med. 163, 238–243.

Pallesen, S., Molde, H., Arnestad, H.M., Laberg, J.C., Skutle, A., Iversen, E., et al., 2007. Outcome of pharmacological treatments of pathological gambling: A review and meta-analysis. J Clin Psychopharmacol. 27, 357–364.

Perez de Castro, I., Ibanez, A., Torres, P., Saiz-Ruiz, J., Fernandez-Piqueras, J., 1997. Genetic association study between pathological gambling and a functional DNA polymorphism at the D4 receptor gene. Pharmacogenetics. 7, 345–348.

Perez de Castro, I., Ibanez, A., Saiz-Ruiz, J., Fernandez-Piqueras, J., 2002. Concurrent positive association between pathological gambling and functional DNA polymorphisms at the MAO-A and the 5-HT transporter genes. Mol Psychiatry. 7, 927–928.

Peters, J., Bromberg, U., Schneider, S., Brassen, S., Menz, M., Banaschewski, T., et al., IMAGEN Consortium, 2011. Lower ventral striatal activation during reward anticipation in adolescent smokers. Am J Psychiatry. 168, 540–549.

Petry, N.M., 2001. Substance abuse, pathological gambling, and impulsiveness. Drug Alcohol Depend. 63, 29–38.

Petry, N.M., 2003. Patterns and correlates of Gamblers Anonymous attendance in pathological gamblers seeking professional treatment. Addict Behav. 28, 1049–1062.

Petry, N.M., 2005. Gamblers anonymous and cognitive–behavioral therapies for pathological gamblers. J Gambl Stud. 21, 27–33.

Petry, N.M., 2007. Concurrent and predictive validity of the Addiction Severity Index in pathological gamblers. Am J Addict. 16, 272–282.

Petry, N.M., Casarella, T., 1999. Excessive discounting of delayed rewards in substance abusers with gambling problems. Drug Alcohol Depend. 56, 25–32.

Petry, N.M., Armentano, C., Kuoch, T., Norinth, T., Smith, L., 2003. Gambling participation and problems among South East Asian refugees to the United States. Psychiatr Serv. 54, 1142–1148.

Petry, N.M., Stinson, F.S., Grant, B.F., 2005. Comorbidity of DSM-IV pathological gambling and other psychiatric disorders: Results from the National Epidemiologic Survey on Alcohol and Related Conditions. J Clin Psychiatry. 66, 564–574.

Petry, N.M., Weinstock, J., Ledgerwood, D.M., Morasco, B., 2008. A randomized trial of brief interventions for problem and pathological gamblers. J Consult Clin Psychol. 76, 318–328.

Petry, N.M., Weinstock, J., Morasco, B.J., Ledgerwood, D.M., 2009. Brief motivational interventions for college student problem gamblers. Addiction. 104, 1569–1578.

Petry, N.M., Blanco, C., Stinchfield, R., Volberg, R., 2013. An empirical evaluation of proposed changes for gambling diagnosis in the DSM-5. Addiction. 108, 575–581.

Reuter, J., Raedler, T., Rose, M., Hand, I., Glascher, J., Buchel, C., 2005. Pathological gambling is linked to reduced activation of the mesolimbic reward system. Nat Neurosci. 8, 147–148.

Rush, B.R., Bassani, D.G., Urbanoski, K.A., Castel, S., 2008. Influence of co-occurring mental and substance use disorders on the prevalence of problem gambling in Canada. Addiction. 103, 1847–1856.

Saiz-Ruiz, J., Blanco, C., Ibanez, A., Masramon, X., Gomez, M.M., Madrigal, M., et al., 2005. Sertraline treatment of pathological gambling: A pilot study. J Clin Psychiatry. 66, 28–33.

Sescousse, G., Redoute, J., Dreher, J.C., 2010. The architecture of reward value coding in the human orbitofrontal cortex. J Neurosci. 30, 13095–13104.

Sher, K.J., Bartholow, B.D., Wood, M.D., 2000. Personality and substance use disorders: A prospective study. J Consult Clin Psychol. 68, 818–829.

Slutske, W.S., 2006. Natural recovery and treatment-seeking in pathological gambling: Results of two U.S. national surveys. Am J Psychiatry. 163, 297–302.

Slutske, W.S., Eisen, S., True, W.R., Lyons, M.J., Goldberg, J., Tsuang, M., 2000. Common genetic vulnerability for pathological gambling and alcohol dependence in men. Arch Gen Psychiatry. 57, 666–673.

Slutske, W.S., Eisen, S., Xian, H., True, W.R., Lyons, M.J., Goldberg, J., et al., 2001. A twin study of the association between pathological gambling and antisocial personality disorder. J Abnorm Psychol. 110, 297–308.

Slutske, W.S., Caspi, A., Moffitt, T.E., Poulton, R., 2005. Personality and problem gambling: A prospective study of a birth cohort of young adults. Arch Gen Psychiatry. 62, 769–775.

Slutske, W.S., Moffitt, T.E., Poulton, R., Caspi, A., 2012. Undercontrolled temperament at age 3 predicts disordered gambling at age 32: A longitudinal study of a complete birth cohort. Psychol Sci. 23, 510–516.

Stewart, R.M., Brown, R.I., 1988. An outcome study of Gamblers Anonymous. Br J Psychiatry. 152, 284–288.

Stinchfield, R., 2002. Reliability, validity, and classification accuracy of the South Oaks Gambling Screen (SOGS). Addict Behav. 27, 1–19.

Stinchfield, R., 2010. A critical review of adolescent problem gambling assessment instruments. Int J Adolesc Med Health. 22, 77–93.

Strobel, A., Wehr, A., Michel, A., Brocke, B., 1999. Association between the dopamine D4 receptor (DRD4) exon III polymorphism and measures of Novelty Seeking in a German population. Mol Psychiatry. 4, 378–384.

Stucki, S., Rihs-Middel, M., 2007. Prevalence of adult problem and pathological gambling between 2000 and 2005: An update. J Gambl Stud. 23, 245–257.

Toce-Gerstein, M., Gerstein, D.R., Volberg, R.A., 2009. The NODS-CLiP: A rapid screen for adult pathological and problem gambling. J Gambl Stud. 25, 541–555.

Tozzi, L., Akre, C., Fleury-Schubert, A., Suris, J.C., 2013. Gambling among youths in Switzerland and its association with other addictive behaviours: A population-based study. Swiss Med Wkly. 143, w13768.

van Holst, R.J., van den Brink, W., Veltman, D.J., Goudriaan, A.E., 2010. Why gamblers fail to win: A review of cognitive and neuroimaging findings in pathological gambling. Neurosci Biobehav Rev. 34, 87–107.

van Holst, R.J., de Ruiter, M.B., van den Brink, W., Veltman, D.J., Goudriaan, A.E., 2012a. A voxel-based morphometry study comparing problem gamblers, alcohol abusers, and healthy controls. Drug Alcohol Depend. 124, 142–148.

van Holst, R.J., van der Meer, J.N., McLaren, D.G., van den Brink, W., Veltman, D.J., Goudriaan, A.E., 2012b. Interactions between affective and cognitive processing systems in problematic gamblers: A functional connectivity study. PLoS ONE. 7, e49923.

Verdejo-Garcia, A., Lawrence, A.J., Clark, L., 2008. Impulsivity as a vulnerability marker for substance-use disorders: Review of findings from high-risk research, problem gamblers and genetic association studies. Neurosci Biobehav Rev. 32, 777–810.

Villella, C., Martinotti, G., Di Nicola, M., Cassano, M., La Torre, G., Gliubizzi, M.D., et al., 2011. Behavioural addictions in adolescents and young adults: Results from a prevalence study. J Gambl Stud. 27, 203–214.

Vitaro, F., Arseneault, L., Tremblay, R.E., 1999. Impulsivity predicts problem gambling in low SES adolescent males. Addiction. 94, 565–575.

Volberg, R.A., Steadman, H.J., 1989. Prevalence estimates of pathological gambling in New Jersey and Maryland. Am J Psychiatry. 146, 1618–1619.

Volberg, R.A., Abbott, M.W., Ronnberg, S., Munck, I.M., 2001. Prevalence and risks of pathological gambling in Sweden. Acta Psychiatr Scand. 104, 250–256.

Volberg, R.A., Gupta, R., Griffiths, M.D., Olason, D.T., Delfabbro, P., 2010. An international perspective on youth gambling prevalence studies. Int J Adolesc Med Health. 22, 3–38.

Volberg, R.A., Munck, I.M., Petry, N.M., 2011. A quick and simple screening method for pathological and problem gamblers in addiction programs and practices. Am J Addict. 20, 220–227.

Volkow, N.D., Ding, Y.S., Fowler, J.S., Wang, G.J., 1996. Cocaine addiction: Hypothesis derived from imaging studies with PET. J Addict Dis. 15, 55–71.

Volkow, N.D., Wang, G.J., Fowler, J.S., Logan, J., Angrist, B., Hitzemann, R., et al., 1997. Effects of methylphenidate on regional brain glucose metabolism in humans: Relationship to dopamine D2 receptors. Am J Psychiatry. 154, 50–55.

Volkow, N.D., Chang, L., Wang, G.J., Fowler, J.S., Ding, Y.S., Sedler, M., et al., 2001. Low level of brain dopamine D2 receptors in methamphetamine abusers: Association with metabolism in the orbitofrontal cortex. Am J Psychiatry. 158, 2015–2021.

Walther, B., Morgenstern, M., Hanewinkel, R., 2012. Co-occurrence of addictive behaviours: Personality factors related to substance use, gambling and computer gaming. Eur Addict Res. 18, 167–174.

Wardman, D., el-Guebaly, N., Hodgins, D., 2001. Problem and pathological gambling in North American Aboriginal populations: A review of the empirical literature. J Gambl Stud. 17, 81–100.

Welte, J., Barnes, G., Wieczorek, W., Tidwell, M.C., Parker, J., 2001. Alcohol and gambling pathology among U.S. adults: Prevalence, demographic patterns and comorbidity. J Stud Alcohol. 62, 706–712.

White, M.J., Young, R.M., Morris, C.P., Lawford, B.R., 2011. Cigarette smoking in young adults: The influence of the HTR2A T102C polymorphism and punishment sensitivity. Drug Alcohol Depend. 114, 140–146.

Wickwire, E.M., Burke, R.S., Brown, S.A., Parker, J.D., May, R.K., 2008. Psychometric evaluation of the National Opinion Research Center DSM-IV Screen for Gambling Problems (NODS). Am J Addict. 17, 392–395.

Wilson, D., da Silva Lobo, D.S., Tavares, H., Gentil, V., Vallada, H., 2013. Family-based association analysis of serotonin genes in pathological gambling disorder: Evidence of vulnerability risk in the 5HT-2A receptor gene. J Mol Neurosci. 49, 550–553.

Winters, K.C., Rich, T., 1998. A twin study of adult gambling behavior. J Gambl Stud. 14, 213–225.

Wise, R.A., 2004. Dopamine, learning and motivation. Nat Rev Neurosci. 5, 483–494.

Wong, I.L., So, E.M., 2003. Prevalence estimates of problem and pathological gambling in Hong Kong. Am J Psychiatry. 160, 1353–1354.

Wulfert, E., Hartley, J., Lee, M., Wang, N., Franco, C., Sodano, R., 2005. Gambling screens: Does shortening the time frame affect their psychometric properties? J Gambl Stud. 21, 521–536.

Zucker, R.A., 2008. Anticipating problem alcohol use developmentally from childhood into middle adulthood: What have we learned? Addiction. 103(Suppl 1), 100–108.

3

Internet Gaming Disorder

A New Behavioral Addiction

**FLORIAN REHBEIN, SIMONE KÜHN,
HANS-JÜRGEN RUMPF, AND NANCY M. PETRY** ■

Internet gaming disorder, which is also referred to as video game addiction, pathological gaming, and a variety of other terms, was included in the fifth edition of the *Diagnostic and Statistical Manual of Mental Disorders* (DSM-5) in Section 3, Conditions for Further Study. This chapter describes the DSM-5 classification system for Internet gaming disorder, as well as the general concept of this proposed disorder and its distinction from other conditions, particularly Internet addiction and gambling disorder. The chapter also describes international prevalence rates of Internet gaming disorder and comorbidities between gaming disorder and other psychiatric conditions. In addition, the chapter outlines risk and protective factors, including demographic and social, game-related, psychological, neurophysiological, and genetic risk factors. Finally, the chapter summarizes the limited research on treatment of the disorder and discusses future research directions to improve the diagnosis, prevention, and treatment of this behavioral addiction.

DEFINING FEATURES AND METHODS FOR ASSESSMENT

Excessive use of video and computer games is a frequent phenomenon, particularly in male adolescents. However, spending substantial time playing games alone is not a sufficient indicator of clinical distress or a psychiatric condition. Although most people who are "addicted" to video games play for considerably long periods of time, the reverse is not necessarily true. Only a proportion of excessive gamers also exhibit psychological symptoms that warrant a possible psychiatric diagnosis of Internet gaming disorder. One criterion that distinguishes those with a problem with gaming from those without is that those with a problem play video games not just for fun but also to forget about real-life problems and manage negative emotions. Problem gamers' thoughts and behaviors become increasingly more constricted to gaming, resulting in adverse effects on social and functional areas of life. Another characteristic feature is loss of control, which prevents gamers from regulating the frequency and intensity of their gaming activities. In particularly serious cases, severe hazards and losses may result, such as dropping out of school, losing one's job, and breaking up with a partner (Beutel et al., 2011). In some cases, extreme and incessant gaming has been reported to lead to serious health problems, such as strokes (Chuang, 2006) and death (BBC News, 2005; Reuters, 2007).

It is important to distinguish Internet gaming disorder from two other disorders, which will be addressed in other sections of this book: Internet addiction and gambling disorder. The term *Internet addiction* refers to adverse consequences arising from any activity that can be performed online (Young et al., 1999), whereas the term *Internet gaming disorder* focuses exclusively on the excessive and problematic usage of video or computer games. The disorder is intended to cover electronic games played online or offline, and accordingly, Internet gaming disorder constitutes a separate nosological entity that does not fully overlap with Internet addiction (Rehbein and Mößle, 2013).

Another important distinction must be made in regard to gambling disorder. *Gambling disorder* refers to excessive and problematic participation in games in which one risks money or items of monetary value in hopes of a larger financial payout. These are not primary characteristics of video games. In some video games, players can unlock items that have an actual monetary value and can be sold for real money, but the primary purpose of playing is not for financial gain, and money is not risked. Gaming and gambling also differ with respect to the factors that influence the player's success; video game playing is primarily skill dependent, whereas the results of many gambling activities are influenced only to a limited degree (e.g., in the case of sports betting and some card games) or not at all (e.g., in the case of lotteries, roulette, and slot machines) by knowledge or skill (Meyer and Bachmann, 2011).[1]

Following the recommendation of the substance use disorder (SUD) workgroup of the DSM-5, gambling disorder was the first non-substance addictive-related behavior to be included in the DSM-5 chapter "Substance-Related and Addictive Disorders." This decision was based on epidemiological, biological, and conceptual similarities between gambling and substance-related disorders (Petry and O'Brien, 2013; Petry et al., 2014). Internet gaming disorder was the only other non-substance addiction included and was listed in Section 3 of the DSM-5, "Conditions for Further Study" (American Psychiatric Association, 2013). The SUD workgroup concluded that a growing body of evidence existed regarding the risk of clinically significant impairment in individuals with Internet gaming disorder, but there still was not sufficient data to support specific criteria for diagnosis of a mental disorder related to game playing. The workgroup noted that no standard diagnostic criteria existed, and the assessment tools and cutoff values varied considerably across studies (Petry et al., 2014). The inclusion of this condition in Section 3 of the DSM-5 was intended to stimulate further research in this area.

The DSM-5 lists nine possible criteria for Internet gaming disorder:

1. Preoccupation with games (i.e., "cognitive salience")
2. Withdrawal symptoms when gaming is not possible
3. Tolerance—the need to spend increasing amounts of time engaged in games
4. Unsuccessful attempts to control participation in games
5. Loss of interest in previous hobbies and entertainment as a result of, and with the exception of, games (i.e., "behavioral salience")

6. Continued excessive use of games despite knowledge of psychosocial problems
7. Deceit of family members, therapists, or others regarding the amount of gaming
8. Use of games to escape or relieve a negative mood
9. Risk or loss of a significant relationship, job, or educational or career opportunity because of participation in games

The DSM-5 suggested a conservative cut-point of endorsing at least five of nine criteria in the past 12 months for diagnosis. This threshold is intended to prevent overdiagnosis (Petry et al., 2014). Only problems associated with the use of video and computer games are considered. As stated explicitly in the DSM-5, the diagnosis is intended to cover both online games (games that are played on the Internet) and offline games (games that are played without an active Internet connection), even though the word "Internet" is included in the title (primarily to distinguish gaming disorder from gambling disorder). However, the diagnosis is not intended to be applied to other types of Internet or computer usage including online gambling, which falls into the category of gambling disorder (see Chapter 2).

The DSM-5 establishes the first standard for classification of Internet gaming disorder. However, the criteria and cut-point suggested may not accurately represent a disorder, and they require further study. The lack of consensus related to operationalization of the criteria is illustrated by examination of existing tools that intend to characterize criteria. Close inspection of wording of criteria in these instruments reveals large discrepancies in their interpretation (Petry et al., 2014).

A publication of an international group of authors—including four members of the DSM-5 SUD workgroup—provides suggestions for more consistent interpretation of the Internet gaming disorder criteria (Petry et al., 2014). The authors argue that criterion 1 (cognitive preoccupation) must focus on periods of time in which the person is not playing videos games. Furthermore, the thoughts have to recur several times in the course of a day. Regarding criterion 2 (withdrawal),

withdrawal symptoms have to occur in those situations in which the person does not have the opportunity to play video games or attempts to stop playing. It is essential not to mistake immediate intense emotions that result from an external interference for withdrawal symptoms (e.g., an adolescent's tantrum when the game console is deactivated by his or her parents). Concerning criterion 3 (tolerance), an increase in gaming times (which may result from various factors, such as having more leisure time) does not necessarily indicate the development of tolerance. Rather, an increase in gaming must be the consequence of a growing desire for video gaming or more exciting gaming experiences. In terms of criterion 4 (unsuccessful attempts to control), the loss of control has to be significant enough to include unsuccessful efforts to cut down gaming, thus indicating a tendency to relapse. Regarding criterion 5 (loss of interests), the constriction of behavior must include a loss of interest in other activities as well as a considerable reduction of other activities to spend more time with gaming. In the discussion of criterion 6 (excessive gaming despite problems), several characteristics of psychosocial problems are highlighted, including prolonged and clinically significant aspects of central functioning, not simply mild and transient consequences such as sleeping less when it does not interfere with functioning. The authors argue that criterion 7 (deception) covers both lying and attempts to conceal gaming activities. The dysfunctional usage of video games addressed in criterion 8 (escape or relief from a negative mood) requires gaming to be engaged in as a way of forgetting real-life problems or relieving dysphoric emotions, but only emotions not reflecting withdrawal symptoms are relevant to this criterion. Criterion 9 (jeopardized or lost) is a particularly severe criterion because it refers to the occurrence of damages in social (jeopardizing or losing significant relationships) or performance-related spheres (losing one's job and jeopardizing career or educational opportunities).

Many classification systems that have been applied to assess Internet gaming disorder were developed for the assessment of Internet addiction more globally (Beard and Wolf, 2001; Ko et al., 2005b; Young, 1998) and then applied to gaming (Gentile, 2009; Lemmens et al., 2009; Pápay et al., 2013; Rehbein et al., 2009; Sim et al., 2012; Wölfling et al., 2008, 2011). The existing tools do not fully encompass the nine DSM-5 criteria, although there is some overlap. In particularly, the first six DSM-5 criteria of Internet gaming disorder are addressed by most, but certainly not all, screening instruments (Rehbein and Mößle, 2012). In contrast, criteria 7 to 9 were rarely, or only partially, covered in most instruments. As the field progresses, it will be critical to revise and adapt existing instruments for both screening and diagnostic purposes.

Ko and colleagues (2014) administered clinical interviews based on the DSM-5 Internet gaming disorder criteria to three subgroups of individuals: those with current gaming problems, those with past but not current gaming problems, and a control group. Their results indicated that criteria 6, "continuation despite problems," and 9, "losses," had high diagnostic accuracy in discriminating between the control and gaming disorder groups, whereas criterion 7, "deception," had the lowest diagnostic accuracy (Ko et al., 2014). They also assessed different cut-points for classification and determined that meeting five or more DSM-5 criteria resulted in the best diagnostic accuracy in terms of distinguishing individuals with "normal" levels of play from those who had experienced clinically significant harms from game playing. This study represents the first attempt at applying the DSM-5 criteria in the context of a diagnostic interview. Additional work will be needed to evaluate these criteria in the context of structured interviews in other samples and cultures. Finally, brief screening tools require development for use in population or epidemiological samples.

PREVALENCE RATES

Although no established screening tool exists to classify Internet gaming disorder as described in the DSM-5, a number of epidemiological studies have been conducted to estimate the prevalence of gaming problems in the general population. Eight studies involving large sample sizes and random sampling procedures are published. Four of these studies were conducted in Germany (Festl et al., 2013; Mößle, 2012; Rehbein et al., 2010; Schmidt et al., 2011). The remaining four are from Norwegian (Mentzoni et al., 2011), U.S. (Gentile, 2009), Hungarian (Pápay et al., 2013), and Australian samples (King et al., 2013). Five of the studies targeted adolescents, whereas the other three studies focused on a larger age range and included adult subjects. Table 3.1 provides an overview of these eight studies.

To assess addictive video game play, all studies used short questionnaires. Three used the Video Game Dependency Scale (CSAS-II; Rehbein et al., 2010), two used the Game Addiction Scale (GASA; Lemmens et al., 2009), and one study each utilized the Pathological Gaming Scale (PGS; Gentile, 2009), the Problematic Online Gaming Questionnaire (POGQ-SF; Pápay et al., 2013), and the Pathological Technology Use checklist (PTU; Sim et al., 2012). Each of these instruments has limitations as described previously, and none evaluated all of the DSM-5 criteria.

The prevalence rates derived from these studies varied rather vastly, in part because of the different instruments applied and criteria assessed to classify gaming addition. The U.S. study, for example, found that 8.5% of children and adolescents aged 8 to 18 years exhibit "pathological gaming" (Gentile, 2009). This relatively high prevalence rate may reflect that the instrument classified persons as addicted when the consequences of game playing were not clinically severe (e.g., neglecting household duties to play). Smaller proportions of adolescents were reported by a Hungarian study, which estimated a prevalence rate of 4.6% (Pápay et al., 2013), and an Australian study with a prevalence of 1.8% (King et al., 2013). German adolescents appear to have prevalence rates ranging from 1.7% to 1.9%. (Mößle, 2012; Rehbein et al., 2010).

Studies investigating the prevalence of Internet gaming disorder in adults are even more limited. Two German studies (Festl et al., 2013; Schmidt et al., 2011) reported that 0.2% to 0.5% of adults in Germany exhibit addictive game playing behavior. A study in Norway reported a prevalence rate of 0.6% for persons aged 15 to 40 years (Mentzoni et al., 2011), comparable to the proportion found in the German study by Schmidt et al. (2011).

Table 3.1 Epidemiological Studies on the Prevalence of Internet Gaming Disorder (2009–2013)

Reference	Country	Sample (N)	Age (Years)	Sample	Sex, Male (%)	Moderate Risk/ Endangered (%)	High Risk/ Pathological (%)	Instrument
Gentile (2009)	United States	1,178	8–18	National	n.s.	8.5 (total)		PGS
Rehbein et al. (2010)	Germany	15,168	$M = 15.3$	National	51	2.8	1.7	CSAS-II
Schmidt et al. (2011)	Germany	600	14–60+	National (gamer)	57	0.9	0.5	CSAS-II
Mentzoni et al. (2011)	Norway	816	15–40	National	62	n.s.	0.6	GASA
Mößle (2012)	Germany	806	$M = 12.5$	Berlin	50	2.1	1.9	CSAS-II
Festl et al. (2013)	Germany	4,382	$M = 37.8$	National (gamer)	58	3.7	0.2	GASA
Pápay et al. (2013)	Hungary	5,045	$M = 16.4$	National (gamer)	51	13.3	4.6	POGQ-SF
King et al. (2013)	Australia	1,287	$M = 14.8$	South Australia	50	n.s.	1.8	PTU

n.s., not specified; M, arithmetic mean; CSAS-II, Video Game Dependency Scale (Rehbein et al., 2010); GASA, Game Addiction Scale for Adolescents (Lemmens et al., 2009); PGS, Pathological Gaming Scale (Gentile, 2009); POGQ-SF, Problematic Online Gaming Questionnaire (Pápay et al., 2013); PTU, Pathological Technology Use checklist (Sim et al., 2012).

However, these estimates should be considered cautiously. gested threshold for diagnosis of five of nine criteria in DSM-5 de creates a conservative standard, intended to prevent an overestir the occurrence of Internet gaming disorder in the general population. It is likely that future studies using DSM-5 standards will report lower prevalence rates than most of the studies conducted to date.

COMORBIDITIES

Individuals with Internet gaming disorder exhibit high overall levels of psychological distress (Beutel et al., 2011; Rehbein et al., 2011; Starcevic et al., 2011). Compared to controls, they also report reduced sleeping time (Achab et al., 2011; Rehbein and Mößle, 2013) and greater difficulties falling asleep (Rehbein and Mößle, 2013).

Depression is the psychological condition that has been most often studied in the context of Internet gaming disorder, and virtually all studies that have assessed depression find an association with Internet gaming disorder (Desai et al., 2010; Gentile et al., 2011; Li et al., 2011; Mentzoni et al., 2011; Metcalf and Pammer, 2011; van Rooij et al., 2011, 2012; Wenzel et al., 2009). Consistent with this association, loneliness (Lemmens et al., 2009, 2011; van Rooij et al., 2001, 2012; Walther et al., 2012) and low life satisfaction (Ko et al., 2005a; Lemmens et al., 2009, 2011; Mentzoni et al., 2011) have been noted in those with Internet gaming disorder compared to those without. Importantly, approximately 43% of girls and 13% of boys with Internet gaming disorder report frequent suicidal thoughts versus only approximately 4% of girls and 2% of boys without the disorder (Rehbein and Mößle, 2013).

Three studies found that attention deficit hyperactivity disorder is associated with Internet gaming disorder in children, adolescents, and young adults (Bioulac et al., 2008; Gentile, 2009; Walther et al., 2012). In addition, there is evidence that individuals with Internet gaming disorder exhibit a high level of anxiety (Gentile et al., 2011; Mentzoni et al., 2011; Metcalf and Pammer, 2011), especially as relates to school (Batthyány et al., 2009;

Rehbein et al., 2010) and social interactions (Gentile et al., 2011; van Rooij et al., 2012; Walther et al., 2012). In two clinical studies, boys with autism spectrum disorder were found to be prone to addictive gaming as well (Mazurek and Engelhardt, 2013; Mazurek and Wenstrup, 2013).

Relatively few studies have investigated the comorbidity of Internet gaming disorder and other behavioral addictions. Two studies point to a possible overlap between Internet gaming disorder and gambling disorder (Parker et al., 2008; Walther et al., 2012). Some studies have examined gaming alongside Internet addiction and indicate high comorbidities between both phenomena. Rehbein and Mößle (2013) reported that 26% of adolescents with Internet gaming disorder appeared to be also addicted to Internet activities excluding gaming. King and colleagues (2013) reported that out of 63 secondary school students fulfilling the criteria of pathological video gaming, 40 (65%) also endorsed similar criteria related to Internet addiction more globally, excluding gaming. However, these particularly high comorbidities may have arisen because of difficulties in separating Internet gaming disorder from other forms of pathological Internet use.

In contrast to other behavioral additions, research on the comorbidity between Internet gaming disorder and other substance-related disorders is virtually unknown. Only in a very few studies has the relationship of Internet gaming disorder to alcohol, nicotine, and caffeine consumption (not addictive use) been analyzed, rendering mixed results, with one study finding an association with a higher rate of smoking (in boys) and drug use (in girls) (Desai et al., 2010) and another study reporting no such association (Walther et al., 2012). Particularly inconclusive are the results regarding caffeine consumption, which was reported to be lower in students with Internet gaming disorder in one study (Desai et al., 2010) and higher in another (Porter et al., 2010). However, these studies are plagued by measurement issues and other methodological concerns that may impact interpretation of the findings.

One study has followed up individuals from a large general population sample (Rumpf et al., 2014a) showing signs of excessive Internet use (21 or more points on the CIUS; Meerkerk et al., 2009) and conducted in-depth personal interviews including psychiatric comorbidity. In those fulfilling at least five DSM-5 criteria of Internet gaming disorder and who reported that gaming was their main activity on the Internet, high proportions of comorbid disorders were found (Rumpf et al., 2014b): substance dependence, 46.7%; mood disorders, 46.7%; anxiety disorders, 23.3%; Cluster A personality disorder, 4.0%; Cluster B personality disorder, 12.0%; and Cluster C personality disorder, 24.0%.

Although cross-sectional research finds associations between Internet gaming disorder and other psychiatric conditions, very little research has been conducted in terms of temporal or causal relationships between other psychiatric conditions and Internet gaming disorder. Initial studies suggest that depression and anxiety may be more likely a consequence, rather than the cause, of Internet gaming disorder among adolescents (Gentile et al., 2011; Mößle and Rehbein, 2013). Nevertheless, reciprocal relationships between Internet gaming disorder and comorbid conditions cannot be ruled out. To clarify these relationships, further longitudinal studies are necessary, especially in high-risk samples, such as those described next.

RISK AND PROTECTIVE FACTORS

Demographic and Social Correlates

The existing studies unanimously find that more males than females are affected by Internet gaming disorder (Mentzoni et al., 2011; Rehbein et al., 2010; Wölfling et al., 2008). The studies also consistently indicate that adolescents develop this condition at higher rates than adults (Mentzoni et al., 2011; Schmidt et al., 2011). In contrast, findings regarding educational background are less consistent. Some studies report higher prevalence rates among people with lower levels of education (Elliott et al., 2012a; Rehbein et al., 2010; Wölfling et al., 2008), whereas others suggest that risk is independent of educational status (Baier and Rehbein, 2009). Further research is needed to shed light on these discrepancies.

In addition to the sociodemographic risk factors, some studies also identified potential social risk factors, especially among children and adolescents. According to the results of one study, ninth-graders with Internet gaming disorder more frequently report a lack of real-life achievements than their counterparts without gaming problems (Rehbein, Kleimann, & Mößle, 2010). Moreover, adolescents seem to be at greater risk if they believe they are poorly integrated into their class at school (Baier and Rehbein, 2009), receive little parental support (Baier and Rehbein, 2009), have parents who frequently play video games (Batthyány et al., 2009), and are being raised in one-parent families (Batthyány et al., 2009).

A few longitudinal studies assessed temporal associations between social risk factors and development of Internet gaming problems. One study suggested that adolescents reporting higher loneliness at the initial assessment period were more likely to develop gaming problems at subsequent assessment periods (Lemmens, Valkenburg, & Peter, 2011). Mößle and Rehbein (2013) found that having difficulties with one's peer group can intensify problematic gaming during the transition from grade 5 to grade 6. Another longitudinal analysis (Rehbein and Baier, 2013) found that 10-year-olds who reported they were raised in one-parent-families, were less integrated in their class at school, and felt less comfortable at school were more likely to exhibit problematic gaming at age 15 years than their counterparts without these characteristics at the age of 10 years. A longitudinal study investigating children and adolescents in Singapore indicated that high parent–child closeness was associated with significant reductions in the number of pathological gaming symptoms over time and that this effect was especially pronounced in boys (Choo et al., 2014).

Game-Related Correlates

Various platforms can be utilized to play games, such as personal computers, game consoles, and mobile gaming devices, and all can lead to problems with gaming. The time spent playing online games is more strongly associated with Internet gaming disorder than time spent playing offline games (Rehbein et al., 2010; Rehbein and Mößle, 2013; Schmidt et al., 2011). However, due to a lack of studies, it is unknown if the platforms and especially mobile versus stationary gaming systems differ with respect to their risk potential. In addition, players can chose from many different types of video games. Two types of games that are often associated with problematic usage are massively multiplayer online role-play games (MMORPGs) and first-person shooters, whereas other types of games, especially those that are often played offline, less often lead to difficulties (Batthyány et al., 2009; Elliott et al., 2012a, 2012b; Mößle and Rehbein, 2013; Rehbein et al., 2010; Smyth, 2007). Thus, the risks associated with particular video games appear to be influenced by structural characteristics of the games, with more active and complex game genres, involving ever-changing virtual worlds and online relationships, more often leading to difficulties. However, the existing research does not yet permit an evaluation of the relevance of specific game characteristics to development of problems, and it remains unclear whether the risk potential of a video game can be inferred from characteristics such as the type of reward allocation or specific features of the virtual environment (Elliott et al., 2012a; King et al., 2010, 2011a).

The players' motivations for playing may also impact development of problems. According to both quantitative and qualitative studies, those with difficulties tend to intensify their playing when they face failures in real-life situations, perhaps suggesting that their gaming behavior relates to an attempt to escape from reality (Batthyány et al., 2009; Grüsser et al., 2005; Hussain and Griffiths, 2009; Kwon et al., 2011; Li et al., 2011; Mößle, 2012; Mößle and Rehbein, 2013; Rehbein et al., 2010; Wan and Chiou, 2006; Wölfling et al., 2008; Zanetta Dauriat et al., 2011).

Personality Factors

Several personality characteristics may also relate to development of Internet gaming disorder. Persons who are addicted to video games exhibit higher impulsivity (Collins et al., 2012; Han et al., 2012b; Liau et al., 2011;

Park et al., 2010; Rehbein et al., 2010; Walther et al., 2012) as well as lower self-esteem (Ko et al., 2005a; van Rooij et al., 2011, 2012) compared to those who do not have gaming problems. Furthermore, studies suggest that individuals with problems related to video game playing display less social competence (Festl et al., 2013; Lemmens et al., 2009; Rehbein et al., 2010), higher levels of physical aggressiveness (Kim et al., 2008; Lemmens et al., 2009; Mehroof and Griffiths, 2010), and less empathy (Parker et al., 2008). Longitudinal studies suggest that high impulsivity, low capacity for empathy, and low social competence predict later development of Internet gaming disorder (Gentile et al., 2011; Lemmens et al., 2011; Mößle and Rehbein, 2013). However, replication of these results is needed before firm conclusions can be drawn regarding these associations.

Neurobiological Risk Factors

Studies have begun to explore structural and functional neural correlates of problematic game playing. Two studies implicate gray matter deficits in the orbitofrontal cortex (OFC). One reported lower gray matter volume in the right OFC (Weng et al., 2013), whereas another found decreases in left lateral OFC thickness (Yuan et al., 2013a). Anatomically, the OFC is a heterogeneous region that has connections with other prefrontal, limbic, sensory, and premotor areas (Öngür and Price, 2000) and is linked to the mesolimbic dopamine system critical for drug reward (Koob and Bloom, 1988). Frontal lobe dysfunction has been associated with a lack of impulse control, greater discounting of delayed rewards, and risky decision-making (Bechara and Van der Linden, 2005). Moreover, impulsiveness is inversely related to OFC volume (Matsuo et al., 2009).

Another brain region implicated in Internet gaming disorder is the bilateral insula (Weng et al., 2013; Yuan et al., 2013a). The insula integrates interoceptive (i.e., bodily) states into conscious feelings and decision-making processes that involve uncertain risk and reward (Verdejo-Garcia et al., 2012). The insula appears to play a role in the decision to take drugs (Naqvi and Bechara, 2009). Weng and colleagues (2013) observed a negative correlation between right OFC and bilateral insula gray matter atrophy and scores on Young's Internet Addiction Scale, indicating that the structural alterations may be associated with the severity of problems.

One study found an increase of gray matter volume associated with Internet gaming disorder in the thalamus (Han et al., 2012b). Another reported an increase in fractional anisotropy of the thalamus, a measure of white matter integrity that was also correlated with the severity of problems (Dong et al., 2012a). The thalamus is involved with reactions to both natural rewards and drugs of abuse (Matzeu et al., 2014). Deficits in brain regions related to sensorimotor coordination such as the cerebellum and inferior parietal lobule have also been reported (Dong et al., 2012b), along with enhanced activation in motor areas (Yuan et al., 2013b) in those with Internet gaming disorder compared to healthy controls. However, because the existing studies are cross sectional in nature, one cannot determine whether the changes observed are a consequence of excessive video gaming or if they predate the onset and increase the likelihood of developing gaming problems.

Several studies compared activity in brain regions using functional magnetic resonance imaging techniques in individuals with Internet gaming disorder and healthy control subjects. The most commonly used task is a cue-induced craving paradigm, in which participants are shown stimuli associated with video games to investigate how the brain responds to them. Most of the studies find that differences between patients and controls resemble those observed in substance use disorders (Ko et al., 2009, 2013a), including enhanced activation in the prefrontal cortex during game-related cues (Ko et al., 2009; Lorenz et al., 2013; Sun et al., 2012). However, the exact location of the between-group differences varies, with changes reported in the OFC (Ko et al., 2009), medial (Lorenz et al., 2013) and lateral frontal cortex (Dong et al., 2013; Ko et al., 2013b), hippocampus and parahippocampus (Ko et al., 2013a; Sun et al., 2012), as well as anterior cingulate cortex (Ko et al., 2009, 2013a; Lorenz et al., 2013). The prefrontal cortex has been associated with appetitive motivation more broadly and with approach toward drug cues more specifically

(Zinser et al., 1999). Some studies also report increased activity during gaming cues in the basal ganglia, particularly in caudate nucleus and nucleus accumbens (Ko et al., 2009; Sun et al., 2012). These brain regions have been related to reward processing and cue reactivity in drugs of abuse (Kühn and Gallinat, 2011). Thus, preliminary research suggests similarities between Internet gaming disorder and substance use disorders in terms of the brain mechanisms underlying these addictive behavioral patterns.

Genetics

In contrast to the growing literature on the neurobiology of Internet gaming disorder, very little research exists on the genetics of this disorder. One study reported that adolescents with Internet gaming disorder had a higher prevalence of the Taq1A1 allele of the dopamine D2 receptor (DRD2 Taq1A1) and the low-activity allele Val158Met in the catecholamine-O-methyltransferase (COMT) genes compared to a healthy control group (Han et al., 2007). The dopamine system is known to be involved in reinforcement and learning, as well as substance dependence (Yacubian and Büchel, 2009). COMT catabolizes dopamine and is important for regulating dopamine levels in the prefrontal cortex, with some evidence linking this gene to addiction as well (Tunbridge et al., 2012). Additional research is needed to confirm and extend these findings to ascertain whether Internet gaming disorder runs in family and has a genetic component and also whether these associations relate to other substance-related and addictive disorders.

TREATMENTS

Because of the nascent nature of Internet gaming disorder, little information is available regarding its treatment. Due to its putative overlap with other behavioral addictions, similar therapeutic approaches have been applied to treat Internet gaming disorder as have been used for treating other addictions. These approaches often aim to enhance the patients' motivation to reduce or stop gaming, address cognitive and behavioral factors that may impact playing, and increase social competence (Mann et al., 2012).

Specialized counseling and treatment programs are available in several countries, although most of these programs address Internet addiction more globally. In particular, many Southeast Asian countries and especially South Korea have established widely publicized Internet addiction treatment facilities (Kim, 2008; King et al., 2011b; Koo et al., 2011). For example, South Korea built up a network of 140 Internet addiction counseling centers and treatment programs at almost 100 hospitals (Kim, 2008). They also initialized the Internet addiction boot camp program called the Jump Up Internet Rescue School (Koo et al., 2011). The program provides a multicomponent eclectic approach toward treatment and restricts computer usage during individuals' stay, which typically lasts 12 days (Koo et al., 2011). No evidence of their efficacy is available, and research related to the short- and long-term benefits of these programs is necessary.

At the Chung Ang University in Seoul, a 3-week brief family therapy intervention was evaluated in a group of 15 adolescents from dysfunctional families also suffering from online game addiction (Han et al., 2012a). The intervention focused on strengthening family cohesion. In response to the therapy, the treatment group of adolescents demonstrated a significant decrease in symptom severity and gaming time, as well as increased activation of the caudate nucleus in response to family affection stimuli (positive family interactions) and decreased activation of dorsolateral prefrontal cortex in response to online game stimuli (Han et al., 2012a). However, due to the small number of subjects, lack of a control condition, and no longer-term follow-up, these results must be considered preliminary at best.

A German outpatient clinic for behavioral addictions provides short-term treatment of Internet and computer game addiction (STICA) (Jäger et al., 2012; Wölfling et al., 2012). STICA combines group with individual therapy for 23 therapy sessions over 4 months. The treatment uses cognitive and behavioral techniques to address reasons for dysfunctional media use by collecting daily diaries of use and analyzing triggers to Internet and gaming use. In addition, social skills training and relapse prevention are provided. The design of a clinical trial evaluating the efficacy of this approach is available (Jäger et al., 2012). The study is ongoing, so no results are available.

Overall, few data exist regarding the efficacy of different treatment approaches for Internet gaming disorder. The majority of publications focus on description of interventions, often borrowed from treatment of substance use and gambling disorders, without providing evidence for their efficacy. A summary of existing reports suggests that treatment may reduce time spent online as well as depressive symptoms (Winkler et al., 2013). Nevertheless, no well-controlled clinical trials of treatment of Internet gaming disorder exist, precluding recommendations of any particular type or focus of treatment at this time.

FUTURE DIRECTIONS

Internet gaming disorder refers to a constellation of symptoms that can arise in response to excessive gaming behavior. The inclusion of Internet gaming disorder in Section 3 of the DSM-5 is a major advance, allowing researchers and clinicians throughout the world a uniform direction to follow when studying and treating this condition. Henceforth, development of psychometrically sound clinical interviews and brief screening tools is necessary. To be compatible with the DSM-5, the diagnostic tools must (1) reflect meaning of the nine criteria of Internet gaming disorder as accurately as possible in a comprehensible manner to youth, (2) capture online as well as offline gaming behavior but not other computer or Internet activities, (3) address clinically significant criteria occurring in a 12-month period, and (4) allow for a categorical diagnostic decision based on the number of diagnostic criteria fulfilled (American Psychiatric Association, 2013; Petry and O'Brien, 2013; Petry et al., 2014).

Other criteria not reflected in the DSM-5 could also be addressed, but at a minimum, it is essential to include the same standard set of criteria. Once specific criteria defining the disorder are established, the frequencies of occurrence of the symptoms can be addressed because some symptoms may need to only occur once, whereas others may need to occur repeatedly, to be associated with harm. A lower cut-point than five criteria may better classify the syndrome if clinically significant symptoms are being addressed. As with other psychiatric disorders, the overall severity of Internet gaming disorder may be distinguished based on symptom counts reflecting mild, moderate, and severe states.

Once psychometrically sound tools are developed, large-scale epidemiological surveys are needed to determine 12-month as well as lifetime prevalence rates of this condition. Studies conducted across cultures and age groups are needed to ensure that similar and clinically relevant constructs are being evaluated. As noted previously, the prevalence rates of the condition vary considerably across studies, primarily due to the heterogeneous approaches applied toward assessment. Cross-cultural and cross-study differences may be much less pronounced if similar assessment approaches were applied.

Another important issue to address is the association of Internet gaming disorder with other psychiatric conditions. In particular, little research to date has evaluated comorbidities of Internet gaming disorder with gambling disorder and substance use disorders, and greater knowledge about these associations is critical to the eventual classification of these conditions under the same rubric (i.e., behavioral addictions). Data related to these issues is relevant not only for the nosological classification of Internet gaming disorder but also for differential diagnosis. In addition, further examination of the neurobiological and genetic underpinnings of Internet gaming disorder and other behavioral addictions will advance the study of all these disorders.

Longitudinal studies are required to understand the natural course of Internet gaming disorder, the risk factors involved in its genesis, as well as the persistence or recovery of symptoms, both with and without treatment. Better knowledge about the course of the condition will be important to guide both prevention and treatment efforts. To date, prevention and early intervention of Internet gaming disorder have rarely been addressed. Given rapidly developing technological advancements in the field of computer and video games (more powerful gaming consoles and computers, increasing relevance of complex online games, and new technologies such as virtual-reality head-mounted displays and innovative input devices), prevention of Internet gaming disorder is of upmost concern.

In summary, research on Internet gaming disorders is in the early stages. However, the growing evidence of clinically significant harms derived from excessive game playing suggests that it is an important area for future research. Much is likely to be learned about this condition in the upcoming years. As a better understanding of this condition is developed, prevention efforts can be aimed particularly at high-risk individuals to minimize the harms of electronic games.

ACKNOWLEDGMENTS

The authors thank Lisa Rothenhöfer and Eva-Maria Zenses for their help in translations and literature research.

NOTE

1. This distinction is becoming less applicable. Complex video games include diverse interactions and unpredictable factors, which weaken the link between the player's skills and the game's outcomes. Consequently, some computer games are becoming more alike to gambling in regard to the random nature of the events and outcomes.

REFERENCES

Achab, S., Nicollier, M., Mauny, F., Monnin, J., Trojak, B., Vandel, P., et al., 2011. Massively multiplayer online role-playing games: Comparing characteristics of addict vs. non-addict online recruited gamers in a French adult population. BMC Psychiatry. 11, 144–154.

American Psychiatric Association, 2013. Diagnostic and statistical manual of mental disorders (5th ed.). Washington, DC: American Psychiatric Association.

Baier, D., Rehbein, F., 2009. Computerspielabhängigkeit im Jugendalter [Video game addiction in adolescence]. In: Tully, C.J. (Ed.), Multilokalität und Vernetzung: Beiträge zur technikbasierten Gestaltung jugendlicher Sozialräume [Multilocality and inter-connectedness: Contributions to the technology-based design of adolescents' social spheres] (pp. 139–155). Weinheim, Germany: Juventa Verlag.

Batthyány, D., Müller, K.W., Benker, F., Wölfling, K., 2009. Computerspielverhalten: Klinische Merkmale von Abhängigkeit und Missbrauch bei Jugendlichen [Video gaming behavior: Clinical aspects of addiction and abuse in adolescents]. Wiener Klinische Wochenschrift. 121, 502–509.

BBC News, 2005. South Korean dies after gaming session. http://news.bbc.co.uk/2/hi/technology/4137782.stm; accessed June 2014.

Beard, K.W., Wolf, E.M., 2001. Modification in the proposed diagnostic criteria for Internet addiction. CyberPsychol Behav. 4, 377–383.

Bechara, A., Van der Linden, M., 2005. Decision-making and impulse control after frontal lobe injuries. Curr Opin Neurol. 18, 734–739.

Beutel, M.E., Hoch, C., Wölfling, K., Müller, K.W., 2011. Klinische Merkmale der Computerspiel- und Internetsucht am Beispiel der Inanspruchnehmer einer Spielsuchtambulanz [Clinical aspects of video gaming- and Internet addiction in patients of a gaming addiction outpatient clinic]. Z Psychosom Med Psychother. 57, 77–90.

Bioulac, S., Arfi, L., Bouvard, M.P., 2008. Attention deficit/hyperactivity disorder and video games: A comparative study of hyperactive and control children. Eur Psychiat. 23, 134–141.

Choo, H., Sim, T., Liau, A.K.F., Gentile, D.A., Khoo, A., 2014. Parental influences on pathological symptoms of video-gaming among children and adolescents: A pro-spective study. J Child Fam Stud. 2014, 1–13.

Chuang, Y.C., 2006. Massively multiplayer online role-playing game-induced sei-zures: A neglected health problem in Internet addiction. Cyberpsychol Behav. 9, 51–456.

Collins, E., Freeman, J., Chamarro-Premuzic, T., 2012. Personality traits associated with problematic and non-problematic massively multiplayer online role playing game use. Pers Indiv Differ. 52, 133–138.

Desai, R.A., Krishnan-Sarin, S., Cavallo, D., Potenza, M.N., 2010. Video-gaming among high school students: Health correlates, gender differences, and problematic gaming. Pediatrics. 126, e1414–e1424.

Dong, G., DeVito, E., Huang, J., Du, X., 2012a. Diffusion tensor imaging reveals thalamus and posterior cingulate cortex abnormalities in Internet gaming addicts. J Psychiat Res. 46, 1212–1216.

Dong, G., Huang, J., Du, X., 2012b. Alterations in regional homogeneity of resting-state brain activity in Internet gaming addicts. Behav Brain Funct. 8, 41–52.

Dong, G., Hu, Y., Lin, X., 2013. Reward/punishment sensitivities among Internet addicts: Implications for their addictive behaviors. Prog Neuro-Psychoph. 46, 139–145.

Elliott, L., Golub, A., Ream, G., Dunlap, E., 2012a. Video game genre as a predictor of problem use. Cyberpsychol Behav Soc Netw. 15, 155–161.

Elliott, L., Ream, G., McGinsky, E., Dunlap, E., 2012b. The contribution of game genre and other use patterns to problem video game play among adult video gamers. Int J Ment Health Addict. 10, 948–969.

Festl, R., Scharkow, M., Quandt, T., 2013. Problematic computer game use among adolescents, younger and older adults. Addiction. 108, 592–599.

Gentile, D.A., 2009. Pathological video-game use among youth ages 8 to 18: A national study. Psychol Sci. 20, 594–602.

Gentile, D.A., Choo, H., Liau, A., Sim, T., Li, D., Fung, D., et al., 2011. Pathological video game use among youths: A two-year longitudinal study. Pediatrics. 127, 319–329.

Grüsser, S.M., Thalemann, R., Albrecht, U., Thalemann, C.N., 2005. Exzessive Computernutzung im Kindesalter—Ergebnisse einer psychometrischen Erhebung [Excessive computer usage in childhood: Results of a psychometric study]. Wiener Klinische Wochenschrift. 117, 188–195.

Han, D., Lee, Y., Yang, K., Kim, E., Lyoo, I., Renshaw, P., 2007. Dopamine genes and reward dependence in adolescents with excessive Internet video game play. J Addict Med. 1, 133–138.

Han, D., Kim, S., Lee, Y., Renshaw, P., 2012a. The effect of family therapy on the changes in the severity of on-line game play and brain activity in adolescents with on-line game addiction. Psychiatry Res Neuroimaging. 202, 126–131.

Han, D., Lyoo, I., Renshaw, P., 2012b. Differential regional gray matter volumes in patients with on-line game addiction and professional gamers. J Psychiatr Res. 46, 507–515.

Hussain, Z., Griffiths, M.D., 2009. The attitudes, feelings, and experiences of online gamers: A qualitative analysis. CyberPsychol Behav. 12, 747–753.

Jäger, S., Müller, K.W., Ruckes, C., Wittig, T., Batra, A., Musalek, M., et al., 2012. Effects of a manualized short-term treatment of Internet and computer game addiction (STICA): Study protocol for a randomized controlled trial. Trials. 13, 43.

Kim, E.J., Namkoong, K., Ku, T., Kim, S.J., 2008. The relationship between online game addiction and aggression, self-control and narcissistic personality traits. Eur Psychiat. 23, 212–218.

Kim, J.-U., 2008. The effect of a R/T group counseling program on the Internet addiction level and self-esteem of Internet addiction university students. Int J Reality Therapy. 27, 4–12.

King, D.L., Delfabbro, P.H., Griffiths, M.D., 2010. Video game structural characteristics: A new psychological taxonomy. Int J Mental Health Addict. 8, 90–106.

King, D.L., Delfabbro, P.H., Griffiths, M.D., 2011a. The role of structural characteristics in problematic video game play: An empirical study. Int J Mental Health Addict. 9, 320–333.

King, D.L., Delfabbro, P.H., Griffiths, M.D., Gradisar, M., 2011b. Assessing clinical trials of Internet addiction treatment: A systematic review and CONSORT evaluation. Clin Psychol Rev. 31, 1110–1116.

King, D.L., Delfabbro, P.H., Zwaans, T., Kaptsis, D., 2013. Clinical features and axis I comorbidity of Australian adolescent pathological Internet and video game users. Aust N Z J Psychiatry. 47, 1058–1067.

Ko, C.-H., Yen, J.-Y., Chen, C.-C., Chen, S.-H., Yen, C.-F., 2005a. Gender differences and related factors affecting online gaming addiction among Taiwanese adolescents. J Nerv Mental Dis. 193, 273–277.

Ko, C.-H., Yen, J.-Y., Chen, C.-C., Chen, S.-H., Yen, C.-F., 2005b. Proposed diagnostic criteria of Internet addiction for adolescents. J Nerv Mental Dis. 193, 728–733.

Ko, C.-H., Liu, G.-C., Hsiao, S., Yen, J.-Y., Yang, M.-J., Lin, W.-C., et al., 2009. Brain activities associated with gaming urge of online gaming addiction. J Psychiatr Res. 43, 739–747.

Ko, C.-H., Liu, G.C., Yen, J.Y., Yen, C.F., Chen, C.S., Lin, W.-C., 2013a. The brain activations for both cue-induced gaming urge and smoking craving among subjects comorbid with Internet gaming addiction and nicotine dependence. J Psychiatr Res. 47, 486–493.

Ko, C.-H., Liu, G.-C., Yen, J.-Y., Chen, C.-Y., Yen, C.-F., Chen, C.-S., 2013b. Brain correlates of craving for online gaming under cue exposure in subjects with Internet gaming addiction and in remitted subjects. Addict Biol. 18(3), 559–569.

Ko, C.-H., Yen, J.-Y., Chen, S.-H., Wang, P.-W., Chen, C.-S., Yen, C.-F., 2014. Evaluation of the diagnostic criteria of Internet gaming disorder in the DSM-5 among young adults in Taiwan. J Psychiatr Res. 53, 103–111.

Koo, C., Wati, Y., Lee, C.C., Oh, H.Y., 2011. Internet-addicted kids and South Korean government efforts: Boot-camp case. Cyberpsychol Behav Soc Netw. 14, 391–394.

Koob, G.F., Bloom, F.E., 1988. Cellular and molecular mechanisms of drug dependence. Science. 242, 715–723.

Kühn, S., Gallinat, J., 2011. Common biology of craving across legal and illegal drugs—A quantitative meta-analysis of cue-reactivity brain response. Eur J Neurosci. 33, 1318–1326.

Kwon, J.-H., Chung, C.-S., Lee, J., 2011. The effects of escape from self and interpersonal relationship on the pathological use of internet games. Community Ment Health J. 47, 113–121.

Lemmens, J.S., Valkenburg, P.M., Peter, J., 2009. Development and validation of a game addiction scale for adolescents. Media Psychol. 12, 77–95.

Lemmens, J.S., Valkenburg, P.M., Peter, J., 2011. Psychosocial causes and consequences of pathological gaming. Comput Hum Behav. 27, 144–152.

Li, D., Liau, A., Khoo, A., 2011. Examining the influence of actual-ideal self-discrepancies, depression, and escapism, on pathological gaming among massively multiplayer online adolescent gamers. Cyberpsychol Behav Soc Netw. 14, 535–539.

Liau, A.K., Neo, E.C., Gentile, D.A., Choo, H., Sim, T., Li, D., Khoo, A., 2011. Impulsivity, self-regulation, and pathological video gaming among youth: testing a mediation model. Asia-Pac J Public Health. doi: 10.1177/1010539511429369

Lorenz, R.C., Krüger, J.-K., Neumann, B., Schott, B.H., Kaufmann, C., Heinz, A., et al., 2013. Cue reactivity and its inhibition in pathological computer game players. Addict Biol. 18, 134–146.

Mann, K., Berner, M., Günthner, A., 2012. Suchterkrankungen [Addictive disorders]. In: Berger, M., Hecht, H. (Eds.), Psychische Erkrankungen: Klinik und Therapie [Mental disorders: Clinical aspects and therapy] (pp. 291–346). Munich: Elsevier.

Matsuo, K., Nicoletti, M., Nemoto, K., Hatch, J.P., Peluso, M.A., Nery, F.G., et al., 2009. A voxel-based morphometry study of frontal gray matter correlates of impulsivity. Hum Brain Mapp. 30, 1188–1195.

Matzeu, A., Zamora-Martinez, E.R., Martin-Fardon, R., 2014. The paraventricular nucleus of the thalamus is recruited by both natural rewards and drugs of abuse: Recent evidence of a pivotal role for orexin/hypocretin signaling in this thalamic nucleus in drug-seeking behavior. Front Behav Neurosci. 8, 117.

Mazurek, M.O., Engelhardt, C.R., 2013. Video game use in boys with autism spectrum disorder, ADHD, or typical development. Pediatrics. 132, 260–266.

Mazurek, M.O., Wenstrup, C., 2013. Television, video game and social media use among children with ASD and typically developing siblings. J Autism Dev Disord. 43, 1258–1271.

Meerkerk, G.-J., Van Den Eijnden, R.J.J.M., Vermulst, A.A., Garretsen, H.F.L., 2009. The Compulsive Internet Use Scale (CIUS): Some psychometric properties. CyberPsychol Behav. 12, 1–6.

Mehroof, M., Griffiths, M.D., 2010. Online gaming addiction: The role of sensation seeking, self-control, neuroticism, aggression, state anxiety, and trait anxiety. Cyberpsychol Behav Soc Netw. 13, 313–316.

Mentzoni, R.A., Brunborg, G.S., Molde, H., Myrseth, H., Skouverøe, K.J.M., Hetland, J., et al., 2011. Problematic video game use: Estimated prevalence and associations with mental and physical health. Cyberpsychol Behav Soc Netw. 14, 591–596.

Metcalf, O., Pammer, K., 2011. Attentional bias in excessive massively multiplayer online role-playing gamers using a modified Stroop task. Comp Hum Behav. 27, 1942–1947.

Meyer, G., Bachmann, M., 2011. Spielsucht: Ursachen, Therapie und Prävention von glücksspielbezogenem Suchtverhalten [Gambling addiction: Causes, therapy, and prevention of gambling-related addictive behavior]. Heidelberg: Springer-Verlag.

Mößle, T., 2012. "Dick, dumm, abhängig, gewalttätig?" Problematische Mediennutzungsmuster und ihre Folgen im Kindesalter. Ergebnisse des Berliner Längsschnitt Medien ["Fat, stupid, addicted, violent?" Problematic media usage behavior and its consequences in childhood. Results of the Berlin Longitudinal Study Media]. Baden-Baden, Germany: Nomos-Verlag.

Mößle, T., Rehbein, F., 2013. Predictors of problematic video game usage in childhood and adolescence. Sucht. 59, 153–164.

Naqvi, N.H., Bechara, A., 2009. The hidden island of addiction: The insula. Trends Neurosci. 32, 56–67.

Öngür, D., Price, J.L., 2000. The organization of networks within the orbital and medial prefrontal cortex of rats, monkeys and humans. Cereb Cortex. 10, 206–219.

Pápay, O., Urbán, R., Griffiths, M.D., Nagygyörgy, K., Farkas, J., Kökönyei, G., et al., 2013. Psychometric properties of the problematic online gaming questionnaire short-form and prevalence of problematic online gaming in a national sample of adolescents. Cyberpsychol Behav Soc Netw. 16, 340–348.

Park, H.S., Kim, S.H., Bang, S.A., Yoon, E.J., Cho, S.S., Kim, S.E., 2010. Altered regional cerebral glucose metabolism in Internet game overusers: A 18F-fluorodeoxyglucose positron emission tomography study. CNS Spectr Int J Neuropsych Med. 15, 159–166.

Parker, J.D.A., Taylor, R.N., Eastabrook, J.M., Schell, S.L., Wood, L.M., 2008. Problem gambling in adolescence: Relationships with Internet misuse, gaming abuse and emotional intelligence. Pers Indiv Differ. 45, 174–180.

Petry, N.M., O'Brien, C.P., 2013. Internet gaming disorder and the DSM-5. Addiction. 108, 1186–1187.

Petry, N.M., Rehbein, F., Gentile, D.A., Lemmens, J.S., Rumpf, H.J., Mößle, T., et al., 2014. An international consensus for assessing Internet gaming disorder using the new DSM-5 approach. Addiction. 109, 1399–1406.

Porter, G., Starcevic, V., Berle, D., Fenech, P., 2010. Recognizing problem video game use. Aust N Z J Psychiatry. 44, 120–128.

Rehbein, F., Baier, D., 2013. Family-, media-, and school-related risk factors of video game addiction: A 5-year longitudinal study. J Media Psychol. 25, 118–128.

Rehbein, F., Mößle, T., 2012. Risikofaktoren für Computerspielabhängigkeit: Wer ist gefährdet? [Risk factors for video game addiction: Who is vulnerable?]. Sucht. 58, 391–400.

Rehbein, F., Mößle, T., 2013. Video game addiction and Internet addiction: Is there a need for differentiation? Sucht. 59, 129–142.

Rehbein, F., Kleimann, M., Mößle, T., 2009. Computerspielabhängigkeit im Kindes- und Jugendalter. Empirische Befunde zu Ursachen, Diagnostik und Komorbiditäten unter besonderer Berücksichtigung spielimmanenter Abhängigkeitsmerkmale [Video game addiction in childhood and adolescence. Empirical evidence concerning causes, diagnosis, and comorbidities with a particular focus on game-immanent characteristics of addiction]. Hannover, Germany: KFN.

Rehbein, F., Kleimann, M., Mößle, T., 2010. Prevalence and risk factors of video game dependency in adolescence: Results of a German nationwide survey. Cyberpsychol Behav Soc Netw. 13, 269–277.

Rehbein, F., Mößle, T., Jukschat, N., Zenses, E.-M., 2011. Zur psychosozialen Belastung exzessiver und abhängiger Computerspieler im Jugend- und Erwachsenenalter [Psychosocial strain of excessive and addicted video gamers in adolescence and adulthood]. Suchttherapie. 12, 64–71.

Reuters, 2007. Online addict dies after "marathon" session. http://www.reuters.com/article/2007/02/28/us-china-internet-addiction-idUSPEK26772020070228; accessed June 2014.

Rumpf, H.-J., Vermulst, A., Bischof, A., Kastirke, N., Gürtler, D., Bischof, G., et al., 2014a. Occurence of Internet addiction in a German general population sample: A latent class analysis. Eur Addict Res. 20, 159–166.

Rumpf, H.-J., Bischof, G., Bischof, A., Besser, B., Glorius, S., deBrito, S., et al., 2014b. Applying DSM-5 criteria for Internet gaming disorder to different Internet activities. Lübeck, Germany: Universität zu Lübeck.

Schmidt, J.-H., Drosselmeier, M., Rohde, W., Fritz, J., 2011. Problematische Nutzung und Abhängigkeit von Computerspielen [Problematic use of and addiction to video games]. In: Fritz, J., Lampert, C., Schmidt, J.-H., Witting, T. (Eds.), Kompetenzen und exzessive Nutzung bei Computerspielern: Gefordert, gefördert, gefährdet [Competencies and excessive use among gamers: Challenged, supported, endangered] (pp. 201–251). Berlin: Vistas-Verlag.

Sim, T., Gentile, D.A., Bricolo, F., Serpelloni, G., Gulamoydeen, F., 2012. A conceptual review of research on the pathological use of computers, video games, and the Internet. Int J Mental Health Addict. 10, 748–769.

Smyth, J.M., 2007. Beyond self-selection in video game play: An experimental examination of the consequences of massively multiplayer online role-playing game play. CyberPsychol Behav. 10, 717–721.

Starcevic, V., Berle, D., Porter, G., Fenech, P., 2011. Problem video game use and dimensions of psychopathology. Int J Mental Health Addict. 9, 248–256.

Sun, Y., Ying, H., Seetohul, R.M., Xuemei, W., Ya, Z., Qian, L., et al., 2012. Brain fMRI study of crave induced by cue pictures in online game addicts (male adolescents). Behav Brain Res. 233, 563–576.

Tunbridge, E.M., Huber, A., Farrell, S.M., Stumpenhorst, K., Harrison, P.J., Walton, M.E., 2012. The role of catechol-O-methyltransferase in reward processing and addiction. CNS Neurol Disord Drug Targets. 11, 306–323.

van Rooij, A.J., Schoenmakers, T.M., Vermulst, A.A., van den Eijnden, R.J.J.M., van de Mheen, D., 2011. Online video game addiction: Identification of addicted adolescent gamers. Addiction. 106, 205–212.

van Rooij, A.J., Schoenmakers, T.M., van den Eijnden, R.J.J.M., Vermulst, A.A., van de Mheen, D., 2012. Video game addiction test: Validity and psychometric characteristics. Cyberpsychol Behav Soc Netw. 15, 507–511.

Verdejo-Garcia, A., Clark, L., Dunn, B.D., 2012. The role of interoception in addiction: A critical review. Neurosci Biobehav Rev. 36, 1857–1869.

Walther, B., Morgenstern, M., Hanewinkel, R., 2012. Co-occurrence of addictive behaviours: Personality factors related to substance use, gambling and computer gaming. Eur Addict Res. 18, 167–174.

Wan, C.-S., Chiou, W.B., 2006. Why are adolescents addicted to online-gaming? An interview study in Taiwan. CyberPsychol Behav. 9, 762–766.

Weng, C.-B., Qian, R.-B., Fu, X.-M., Lin, B., Han, X.-P., Niu, C.-S., et al., 2013. Gray matter and white matter abnormalities in online game addiction. Eur J Radiol. 82, 1308–1312.

Wenzel, H.G., Bakken, I.J., Johannsson, A., Oren, A., 2009. Excessive computer game playing among Norwegian adults: Self-reported consequences of playing and association with mental health problems. Psychol Rep. 105, 1237–1247.

Winkler, A., Dörsing, B., Rief, W., Shen, Y., Glombiewski, J.A., 2013. Treatment of Internet addiction: A meta-analysis. Clin Psychol Rev. 33, 317–329.

Wölfling, K., Thalemann, R., Grüsser-Sinopoli, S.M., 2008. Computerspielsucht: Ein psychopathologischer Symptomkomplex im Jugendalter [Computer gaming addiction: A psychopathological complex of symptoms in adolescence]. Psychiatrische Praxis. 35, 226–232.

Wölfling, K., Müller, K.W., Beutel, M.E., 2011. Reliabilität und Validität der Skala zum Computerspielverhalten (CSV-S) [Reliability and validity of a scale for computer gaming behaviour (CSV-S)]. Psychother Psychosom Med Psychol. 61, 216–224.

Wölfling, K., Jo, C., Bengesser, I., Beutel, M.E., Müller, K.W., 2012. Computerspiel- und Internetsucht: Ein kognitiv-behaviorales Behandlungsmanual [Video game addiction and Internet addiction: A cognitive-behavioral treatment manual]. Stuttgart: Kohlhammer.

Yacubian, J., Büchel, C., 2009. The genetic basis of individual differences in reward processing and the link to addictive behavior and social cognition. Neuroscience. 164, 55–71.

Young, K.S., 1998. Internet addiction: The emergence of a new clinical disorder. CyberPsychol Behav. 1, 237–244.

Young, K.S., Pistner, M., O'Mara, J., Buchanan, J., 1999. Cyber disorders: The mental health concern for the new millennium. CyberPsychol Behav. 2, 475–479.

Yuan, K., Cheng, P., Dong, T., Bi, Y., Xing, L., Yu, D., et al., 2013a. Cortical thickness abnormalities in late adolescence with online gaming addiction. PloS One. 8, e53055.

Yuan, K., Jin, C., Cheng, P., Yang, X., Dong, T., Bi, Y., et al., 2013b. Amplitude of low frequency fluctuation abnormalities in adolescents with online gaming addiction. PloS One. 8, e78708.

Zanetta Dauriat, F.Z., Zermatten, A., Billieux, J., Thorens, G., Bondolfi, G., Zullino, D., et al., 2011. Motivations to play specifically predict excessive involvement in massively multiplayer online role-playing games: Evidence from an online survey. Eur Addict Res. 17, 185–189.

Zinser, M.C., Fiore, M.C., Davidson, R.J., Baker, T.B., 1999. Manipulating smoking motivation: Impact on an electrophysiological index of approach motivation. J Abnorm Psychol. 108, 240–254.

4

Internet Addiction

A Future Addictive Disorder?

HANS-JÜRGEN RUMPF, RAN TAO,
FLORIAN REHBEIN, AND NANCY M. PETRY ■

This chapter focuses on the broad concept of Internet addiction (IA). Chapter 3 reviewed the research on Internet gaming disorder (IGD) specifically, but it did not cover excessive use of the Internet for other purposes. The Internet can, and has been, used excessively and problematically for many purposes beyond gaming. This chapter describes issues related to definitions and assessment, psychiatric comorbidities, and risk and protective factors of IA in a general sense. Although treatment research related to IA is still in its infancy, this chapter outlines available treatments, focusing on that applied in the largest treatment facility in China. The chapter concludes with thoughts about ways to move this field forward.

DEFINING FEATURES AND METHODS FOR ASSESSMENT

In early work of the emerging concept of IA, Young et al. (1999) proposed that individuals could develop problems with a variety of activities on the Internet, including the following: cyber-sexual activities, online relationships (e.g., Facebook), shopping, gambling, trading, e-mailing, surfing, and database searches, as well as gaming. Young et al. additionally pointed out that persons most often become addicted to a particular application, which triggers the pathological behavior.

Given the diverse activities that may lead to excessive or addictive Internet use, many researchers have criticized the construct of IA as a disease entity and suggested that problematic Internet use is more likely a symptom of another underlying disorder (Shaffer et al., 2000). Others have argued that different types of IA exist and should be considered distinct disorders, such that excessive online pornography viewing should be considered separately from excessive online gambling, and both should be distinguished from problematic social networking (Davis, 2001). Still others contend that the Internet is only the delivery mechanism (Sim et al., 2012) and not related to the condition per se. In the case of gambling, this distinction is most straightforward. Gambling disorder is now part of the Substance-Related and Addictive Disorders category in the fifth edition of the *Diagnostic and Statistical Manual of Mental Disorders* (DSM-5; American Psychiatric Association, 2013; Petry et al., 2014). Because gambling disorder is already an established psychiatric condition and the types of activities on which individuals with this disorder wager are not distinguished in diagnosis, this chapter does not include gambling online under the rubric of IA. Similarly, IGD is now included in the research appendix of the DSM-5 as a separate entity, and as such, excessive gaming behaviors are considered separately from excessive use of the Internet for other activities to the extent possible in describing the research on IA.

The frameworks for assessing IA primarily consider DSM criteria from substance use or gambling disorders adapted to Internet activities. Young (1998b) proposed the use of eight DSM gambling criteria pertaining to Internet activities, whereas Griffiths (2005) suggested that substance-related and behavioral addictions share common characteristics. His "components model" consists of the following five criteria: salience, mood modification, tolerance, withdrawal, relapse, and conflict (Griffiths, 2005; Kuss et al., 2014b). Other approaches have mixed criteria from gambling and substance use disorders, and still others have applied different criteria entirely (Davis et al., 2002).

Because of the lack of consensus regarding its defining features, inconsistencies in assessments, and concerns about its uniqueness as a psychiatric condition, IA was not included in DSM-5. However, there is substantial overlap between criteria proposed for IGD as defined in DSM-5 and IA more generally. The majority of criteria included in DSM-5 to define IGD are derived from proposals on the broader concept of IA. From China and Korea, Ko et al. (2009b) and Tao et al. (2010) provide data from different populations to justify the selection of criteria and algorithms to define thresholds for diagnosis of IA. Table 4.1 summarizes these approaches.

Ultimately, the DSM-5 criteria proposed for IGD are likely to be studied in the context of IA, and indeed the DSM-5 specifically indicates that research applying the IGD criteria to IA more broadly is needed to advance an understanding of these conditions. However, review of the available research indicates a lack of consensus in the concepts assessed and instruments applied, making cross-study comparisons difficult (Byun et al., 2009; Shaw and Black, 2008). One systematic search of the literature found 14 questionnaires published in English language peer-reviewed journals (Lortie and Guitton, 2013), and another review (Kuss et al., 2014a) identified 21 different IA assessment instruments. Relatively little information on their psychometric properties is available, and most are only used within one country or one region. One example is the Chen Internet Addiction Scale (CIAS) (Chen et al., 2003), which is often used in studies from China. It has been found to have good psychometric properties (Ko et al., 2009b), but it is not, to the best of our knowledge, used often in studies outside Asia. As another example, 3 questionnaires assessing IA are frequently used in German studies, but they are rarely applied elsewhere (Steffen et al., 2012).

As noted previously, Young (1998b) developed an initial questionnaire for IA using the DSM gambling criteria. She proposed a threshold of five or more of eight criteria for diagnosis. An extended version of the Young Diagnostic Questionnaire (YDQ), and one of the most often used instruments, is the Internet Addiction Test (IAT; Young, 1998a), consisting of 20 items rated on a Likert scale. Some data on its psychometric properties have been published. Widyanto and McMurran (2004) found a

Table 4.1 Criteria Proposed to Define Internet Addiction and Overlaps With Internet Gaming Disorder in DSM-5

Criterion	In Tao et al.'s (2010) Proposal	In Ko et al.'s (2009b) Proposal	In DSM-5 Internet Gaming Disorder
	CLINICAL SYMPTOMS		
Preoccupation with Internet activities	Yes	Yes	Yes
Withdrawal	Yes	Yes	Yes
Tolerance	Yes	Yes	Yes
Unsuccessful attempts to stop or reduce	Yes	Yes?	Yes
Recurrent failure to resist impulse to use Internet	No	Yes	No
Use of Internet for a period longer than intended	No	Yes	No
Excessive time spent on Internet activities and leaving the Internet	No	Yes	No
Excessive efforts spent on activities necessary to obtain access to the Internet	No	Yes	No
Loss of interest in other hobbies or activities	Yes	Yes (as functional impairment)	Yes
Continued excessive use despite problems	Yes	Yes	Yes
Deception regarding the amount of Internet use	Examined, but excluded due to low specificity	No	Yes
Escape or relief a negative mood	Yes	No	Yes
Jeopardized or lost relationship, job or educational or career opportunity	Yes (as functional impairment)	No	Yes

	ADDITIONAL CRITERIA		
Impairment	Functional impairments including loss of a significant relationship, job, educational or career opportunities	1. Recurrent Internet use resulting in failure to fulfill major role obligations 2. Important social/recreational activities given up or reduced because of Internet use 3. Recurrent legal problems because of Internet behavior	
Course/time frame	Duration for at least 3 months, with at least 5 hours of non-business/non-academic use/day	Within the same 3-month period	Within a 12-month period
Exclusion	Not better accounted for by psychotic disorder or bipolar I disorder	Not better accounted for by psychotic disorder or bipolar I disorder or other impulse control disorder or paraphilia	No
DIAGNOSTIC ALGORITHM			
Threshold	A. Preoccupation + withdrawal + one other criterion and Time frame and B. Exclusion criterion and C. Impairment criterion and D. Course criterion	A. Six or more criteria and Time frame and B. One or more impairment criteria and C. Exclusion criterion	Five or more criteria and Time frame

six-factor structure consisting of salience, excessive use, neglecting work, anticipation, lack of control, and neglecting social life. Internal consistencies were moderate, ranging from .54 to .82. The factors correlated with each other, and some were associated with time spent on the Internet, as one index of concurrent validity. In a sample of U.S. college students, a two-factor solution ("dependent use" and "excessive use") emerged, explaining 91% of the total variance in responses (Jelenchick et al., 2012). Thus, this instrument, although widely applied, has relatively limited data on its psychometric properties, some of which are conflicting. More data regarding its sensitivity and specificity in predicting clinically significant harms related to excessive Internet use are needed, as well as longitudinal data related to test–retest reliability and predictive validity in the general population and high-risk samples.

In part due to the lack of consensus regarding the condition of IA and expression of its symptoms, other instruments have added to constructs tapped by the IAT. For example, the Chinese Internet Addiction Inventory (CIAI) uses Young's original questions and adds 22 items (Huang et al., 2007), and the Problematic Internet Use Questionnaire adds 10 items (Demetrovics et al., 2008). Factor analyses of both instruments reveal three, albeit diverging, factors. Using item response theory, another study developed a subsequent version consisting of IAT and CIAT items (Zhang and Xin, 2013). In that sample, the CIAT outperformed the IAT with respect to item and test information. The new 20-item scale consists of 15 CIAT and 5 IAT items, and it has demonstrated improvement compared to the original instruments in terms of increased classification consistency. To date, however, it has only been evaluated in one known sample.

The only questionnaire with data on psychometric properties in large general population studies is the Compulsive Internet Use Scale (CIUS; Meerkerk et al., 2009). It contains 14 items that cover core criteria of addictive Internet use: loss of control, preoccupation, conflict, withdrawal, and coping. A stable one-factor solution was found in the original sample (Meerkerk et al., 2009) and replicated in another large general population study (Guertler et al., 2014a), but other indices of its reliability and validity are still lacking. Similarly, data on an appropriate cut-point for "diagnosis" are limited (Guertler et al., 2014b; Rumpf et al., 2014b), which is a concern that extends across all the existing instruments.

Social networking is increasingly suggested as an Internet activity that might lead to addiction (Andreassen and Pallesen, 2014; Kittinger et al., 2012; Kuss and Griffiths, 2011; Rehbein and Mößle, 2013; Rumpf et al., 2014b), and one study developed a questionnaire to assess Facebook addiction specifically. The Bergen Facebook Addiction Scale (Andreassen et al., 2012) comprises six domains: salience, mood modification, tolerance, withdrawal, conflict, and relapse. Eighteen items were selected based on item-total correlations for each of the six domains. This scale showed good internal consistency and test–retest reliability, as well as correlations with other indices of problems. However, like the other instruments, it has only been evaluated for validity in a limited manner. It is also unclear whether different criteria and assessment instruments are needed to address symptoms and problems associated with different forms of excessive Internet use, or if the conditions can be assessed in a more parsimonious approach by a single tool.

In summary, there are several approaches toward classifying, and a plethora of instruments to assess, IA, and many assess somewhat similar constructs. However, none are widely accepted, and psychometric testing remains limited. A consensus on the defining features of IA is necessary to move this field forward. A brief but comprehensive instrument is needed to evaluate the condition with high levels of reliability and validity across general population and high-risk samples.

PREVALENCE RATES

Prevalence rates of IA are difficult to estimate because of the inconsistencies in instruments applied and different thresholds for classification employed. Most of the questionnaires developed to date are screening instruments and, therefore, by definition cannot confer diagnoses. Typically, clinical interviews are needed to confirm positive screens, but to date no gold standard exists for defining or classifying IA, and few of the screening tools have been validated against clinical assessments. Screening tools always suffer from some degree of false negatives and false positives, and these issues can be especially pronounced in conditions that occur at low rates. Furthermore, low specificity of a screening instrument, which is common, can lead to overestimations of prevalence rates (Gambino, 1997; Wurst et al., 2013).

Compounding these issues in the assessment of IA, most of the samples studied to date have not been representative (Byun et al., 2009). Sample selection bias is a major cause of divergent prevalence estimates. Many prevalence estimates of IA are based on convenience samples (e.g., via online surveys) that provide no indications of, or yield very low, response rates and draw from a subset of the most severe population—that is, those who are online regularly, see the survey link, and choose to respond to it (Byun et al., 2009). Other prevalence estimates are based on studies of subpopulations such as students. Because students use the Internet more than the general population, surveying students also leads to an inflated rate relative to the general population. Few studies of IA have been conducted in a representative sample from the general population.

Finally, as alluded to previously, studies use different criteria to define the condition ranging from at risk to problematic, excessive, compulsive, or addictive Internet use. If milder forms are included in determining prevalence, rates will be artificially higher. As one example of the wide range of prevalence rates, a systematic review of surveys of problematic Internet use in U.S. youth ranged from 0% to 26% (Moreno et al., 2011).

Scores if not hundreds of surveys about excessive IA use have been published, and it is counterproductive to review them all, given concerns about reliability and validity of the instruments applied and selection of samples. The following sections focus on some of the largest studies conducted in representative samples of the general population as well as on the specific subsample of students, who appear to be at high risk for IA. For example, a large and representative study from China surveyed 24,013 fourth- to ninth-graders using the YDQ and reported that 6.3% had IA (Y. A. Li et al., 2014). Four national general population studies on IA have also been published, but they used different assessment approaches. Rates of IA ranged from 0.3% in the United States (Aboujaoude et al., 2006) to 1.0% in Norway (Bakken et al., 2009) and Germany (Rumpf et al., 2014b) and 2.1% in another German study (Müller et al., 2014).

An international study of 10 European countries and Israel conducted with 11,956 adolescents (mean age, approximately 15 years) found an overall prevalence rate of 4.4% for IA (Durkee et al., 2012). It used the YDQ (Cox et al., 2014), with affirmative responses to five or more of eight items classifying IA. The highest prevalence was observed in Israel at 11.8%. Among the European countries, IA was lowest in Italy at 1.2% and highest in Slovenia at 5.8%, suggesting potential cross-cultural differences in rates.

One study utilized latent class analysis to classify IA according to responses on the CIUS (Meerkerk et al., 2009) in a large general population sample from Germany (Rumpf et al., 2014b). In the entire sample aged 14 to 64 years, 1% was classified with IA. Percentages were higher in younger age groups, with up to 4% of participants aged 14 to 16 years identified with IA.

The lack of uniformity in study designs makes it difficult to draw definite conclusions about the prevalence rate of IA or cross-cultural comparisons. However, most studies from the general population that included adults found moderate prevalence rates between approximately 1% and 2.4%. Generally, higher prevalence rates are noted when samples are restricted to students and younger populations, and perhaps especially in non-Western European countries.

COMORBIDITIES

Given concerns about the potential overlap of expression of symptoms related to IA and other conditions, evaluation of psychiatric comorbidities is also critical. A number of studies have evaluated the co-occurrence of other psychiatric conditions with IGD, as described in Chapter 3, and IA, as outlined here. A review of this literature (Carli et al., 2013) identified

20 studies, most of which come from Asian countries. Considering all studies that assessed each condition, 100% reported associations of IA with symptoms of attention deficit hyperactivity disorder (ADHD), 75% with depression, 66% with hostility or aggression, 60% with obsessive–compulsive symptoms, and 57% with anxiety. Overall, these associations were higher among males than females. Contrary to expectations and research related to IGD specifically, none of the studies included in this review reported associations between IA and social phobia (Carli et al., 2013).

In one study, individuals from a large general population sample (Rumpf et al., 2014b) who exhibited symptoms of IA as defined by CIUS scores greater than 21 underwent an in-depth personal interview including assessments of psychiatric comorbidity. Participants who met at least five DSM-5 criteria for IGD as applied to all Internet activities were divided into two groups—those who reported that social networks were their primary form of IA and those who reported that activities other than social networking or gaming were their main Internet activity. In these two subgroups, high rates of comorbid psychiatric disorders were found (Rumpf et al., 2014a). For example, substance dependence was noted in 43.3% of those with IA reporting social networks as their primary activity on the Internet and in 54.5% of those reporting other Internet activities, mood disorders in 53.3% and 50.0%, anxiety disorders in 26.7% and 31.8%, Cluster A personality disorder in 16.0% and 4.8%, Cluster B personality disorder in 16.0% and 14.3%, and Cluster C personality disorder in 8.0% and 33.0%, respectively. At least one personality disorder was noted in 28% of participants with IA for whom social networking was the main activity and in 33% among those with other primary Internet activities. These data indicate high rates of psychiatric comorbidity in persons identified with IA, regardless of the primary Internet activity.

Given the high rate of co-occurring mood disorders, suicidal ideation or suicidal attempts might be another concern among persons with IA. In a study of 9,510 students in Taiwan, IA, as measured with the CIAS (Chen et al., 2003), was associated with suicidal ideation and suicidal attempts even after controlling for demographic variables, depression, family support, and self-esteem (Lin et al., 2014).

In general, the relationship of co-occurring mental disorders and IA can be explained by four hypotheses (Ko et al., 2012): (1) The psychiatric disorder leads to or increases symptoms of IA; (2) IA leads to or deteriorates symptoms of the psychiatric disorder; (3) both disorders have shared underlying mechanisms; or (4) comorbidity is overestimated due to study designs, assessment instruments, or other methodological shortcomings.

Of relevance to the first two hypotheses are longitudinal studies, which can tease out the directionality of the conditions. These studies, however, are rare. One study followed a large sample of adolescents from 10 junior high schools in Taiwan over a period of 2 years (Ko et al., 2009a). Among those without IA at the baseline assessment but who screened positive for IA at a later time point, depression, ADHD, social phobia, and hostility were found to be significant predictors of developing IA. Regardless of gender, ADHD and hostility were the strongest predictors. Although this study is informative about the potential risk factors for IA, assessments of the comorbid disorders were based on brief questionnaires and the follow-up period was only 2 years.

A longitudinal study from China evaluated 59 freshman students who developed IA during their first year at the university (Dong et al., 2011). The Symptom Checklist (SCL-90; Derogatis, 1975) evaluated psychiatric symptoms initially and 1 year later. Some domains showed no changes over time and were unrelated to IA: somatization, paranoid ideation, and phobic anxiety. Scores on the obsessive–compulsive dimension were substantially elevated compared to the norm of the SCL-90 at the initial assessment among those who later developed IA, suggesting this dimension may be associated with onset of IA. Finally, scores on a number of dimensions increased significantly during the follow-up period after students developed IA: depression, anxiety, hostility, interpersonal sensitivity, and psychoticism. Thus, these psychiatric symptoms may arise subsequent to IA.

Taken together, psychiatric comorbidity and symptoms are common in persons with IA. The limited evidence from longitudinal studies suggests that some psychiatric disorders may occur prior to the development of IA, and others may result from IA. More research with larger samples and more systematic evaluation of psychiatric conditions and symptoms is necessary to confirm these initial findings. Such research will be critical to better understanding whether IA should be classified as a unique psychiatric condition or if it is an expression of other underlying psychiatric disorders.

RISK AND PROTECTIVE FACTORS

Demographic Correlates

In general, studies have found higher prevalence rates of IA among men compared to women. Shaw and Black (2008) reviewed 11 studies with gender-specific data and found that 6 reported increased rates of IA among males, 2 among females, and 3 no differences. The authors suggested that the potential increased rates in men may relate to their affinities to gaming and pornography viewing. In a large international and predominantly European study (Durkee et al., 2012), five countries had higher estimates of IA among men, five among women, and in one country rates were equal. The female:male ratio may have changed over time with increasing availability of popular types of Internet activities. Although studies are rare (Andreassen and Pallesen, 2014; Kuss and Griffiths, 2011), recent studies show that women tend to become addicted to using social networks such as Facebook more often than do men (Rehbein and Mößle, 2013; Rumpf et al., 2014b). In a German general population study, there were no overall gender differences with respect to IA, but males reported Internet gaming as a main activity and females reported social networking (Rumpf et al., 2014b). With increasing usage of Facebook and other social network sites, rates of IA may equalize among men and women.

In general population studies, a number of demographic risk factors beyond gender have been considered. In a Norwegian study (Bakken et al., 2009), younger age, university-level education, and low income were associated with at-risk Internet use or IA. Being unmarried, living alone, having no job, being a student, and having low income were found as risk factors in a German general population study (Müller et al., 2014). Another German general population study (Rumpf et al., 2014a) found younger age, migration background, and unemployment to be significantly related to IA. Taken together, these studies seem to suggest that younger age and lower socioeconomic status may be risk factors for developing IA.

Personality Factors and Parenting Style

A number of studies have focused on personality traits and their association with IA. Most of these referred to the Big Five theory (McCrae and Costa, 1987), and many used samples of adolescents or students. In a large sample of adolescents from The Netherlands (Kuss et al., 2013b), emotional stability, agreeableness, and conscientiousness reduced the risk of IA, and resourcefulness increased risk. Using a convenience sample of 2,257 students of an English university, Kuss et al. (2013a) found that high neuroticism and low agreeableness were related to IA. Neuroticism has been found to be a risk factor in other studies (Dong et al., 2013; Tsai et al., 2009), as has low agreeableness (Servidio, 2014).

Several studies have found a relationship between low extraversion and IA (Müller et al., 2013; Servidio, 2014; van der Aa et al., 2009; Xiuqin et al., 2010). Furthermore, in a cross-national study including Bulgaria, Germany, Spain, Colombia, China, Taiwan, and Sweden (Sariyska et al., 2014), self-directedness was negatively correlated to IA, consistent with a Korean study showing IA to be related to low self-directedness, low cooperativeness, high harm avoidance, and high self-transcendence (Ha et al., 2007). However, another Korean study found higher scores in self-directedness in those with IA (Cho et al., 2008). After controlling for ADHD, this study also found that higher scores in cooperativeness and lower scores in novelty seeking and self-transcendence were associated with problematic Internet use. Thus, results are not entirely consistent, but most studies find some associations between personality dimensions and IA.

Another topic of interest is whether parenting style impacts IA (Floros and Siomos, 2013; Siomos et al., 2012; Xiuqin et al., 2010). In a retrospective study (Kalaitzaki and Birtchnell, 2014), self-perceived early parenting styles were indirectly related to the development of IA. They differentiated two dimensions: affectionless control (low care and high protection) and optimal parenting (high care and low protection). With respect to perceived father's rearing style, unfavorable parenting on both dimensions was associated with IA through the mediating role of negatively relating with others (poor ability to establish or maintain mutually satisfying relationships). In terms of recollections of mother's rearing style, less optimal parenting was found to relate to IA through the mediating role of sadness in later life. Another study from China (Yao et al., 2014) revealed that perceptions of fathers' rejection and overprotection, as well as mothers' rejection, had a significant impact on developing IA.

In addition, parent–adolescent interactions may relate to IA (Xu et al., 2014). In a large representative sample of 5,122 students from 16 high schools in Shanghai, worse father–adolescent relationship was related to IA; poor mother–adolescent relationships had an even greater impact (Xu et al., 2014).

Thus, findings from studies on personality factors and parental style suggest that the risk of IA increases in disadvantageous settings, consistent with a diathesis–stress model of IA (van der Aa et al., 2009). Personality vulnerabilities, as well as environmental conditions including poor relationships with parents, may interact to affect IA.

Neurobiological Risk Factors

Neurobiological studies provide further evidence of potential vulnerabilities for IA. Studies evaluating structural or functional brain differences in both those with and those without IA may shed light on the biological basis of this condition. Ultimately, they may be useful for distinguishing IA from other psychiatric conditions and someday may assist in diagnosis.

To date, neurobiological studies of IA have been conducted primarily with Internet gamers, not those with IA more globally, although many studies do not clearly specify or distinguish the nature of the Internet activities (e.g., Yuan et al., 2011). Although several studies have demonstrated changes in brains of persons with IA relative to those without, it is unclear whether these differences result from IA or represent predictors of development of IA. Only longitudinal studies conducted before persons become addicted to the Internet can determine whether changes precede or arise from excessive Internet use.

In functional magnetic resonance imaging (fMRI) studies comparing resting states in IA and non-IA controls, increased regional homogeneity was found in a number of brain regions: cerebellum, brain stem, right cingulate gyrus, bilateral parahippocampus, right frontal lobe (rectal gyrus, inferior frontal gyrus, and middle frontal gyrus), left superior frontal gyrus, left precuneus, right postcentral gyrus, right middle occipital gyrus, right inferior temporal gyrus, left superior temporal gyrus, and middle temporal gyrus (Liu et al., 2010). Regional homogeneity can be interpreted as increased activity, and some of the regions involve reward pathways, suggesting that the sensitivity to reward may be increased in persons with IA. In another study (Kim et al., 2011), reduced levels of dopamine D2 receptor availability were noted in areas of the striatum, including the bilateral dorsal caudate and right putamen. Using a go–stop paradigm in another fMRI study, Li and colleagues (B. Li et al., 2014) reported that the indirect frontal–basal ganglia pathway had no effective connectivity in persons with IA.

To localize abnormal white matter regions potentially associated with IA, fractional anisotropy was used in a diffusion tensor imaging study of 17 subjects with IA and 16 controls (Lin et al., 2012). Compared to controls, IA subjects evidenced significantly lower fractional anisotropy throughout the brain, including the orbitofrontal white matter, corpus callosum, cingulum, inferior fronto-occipital fasciculus, corona radiation, and internal and external capsules. Lower fractional anisotropy was related to duration of IA in another study (Yuan et al., 2011). In addition, gray matter abnormalities have been found, with lower density in the left anterior cingulate cortex, left posterior cingulate cortex, left insula, and left lingual gyrus in IA subjects relative to controls (Zhou et al., 2011).

Although neurobiological studies are limited, abnormalities in IA subjects are generally consistent with those found in subjects with substance use disorders (Volkow et al., 2004). Specifically, studies demonstrate increased reward sensitivity and impaired control or inhibition in subjects with IA and substance use disorders relative to controls. However, and as noted previously, these studies are at early stages, and the directionality and specificity of these effects require additional research.

Genetics

Given that IA has only recently been described and no consensus exists regarding its classification, it is not surprising that very little research on the genetics of this condition is available. One study suggests that serotonin transporter genes may play a role in IA (Lee et al., 2008). That study compared 91 male adolescents with excessive Internet use to 75 controls, and it found that the homozygous short allele variant of the serotonin transporter gene (*SS-5HTTLPR*) was more frequent in the group with excessive Internet use; this gene is also related to harm avoidance. No other genetic studies are available. One other study (Zhang et al., 2013) did evaluate serum levels of neurotransmitters in 20 adolescents with IA and 15 controls; no differences were found in serotonin and dopamine levels in peripheral blood, whereas the mean level of norepinephrine was lower in the IA group. Thus, an understanding of the genetics and neurobiology of IA is in its infancy, and without a consistent and valid method of classifying the condition, such studies may be premature.

TREATMENTS

To date, studies on the treatment of IA are limited, and standard accepted clinical treatment protocols do not exist (Camardese et al., 2012). There is a growing demand for evidence-based recommendations for treatment of all psychiatric conditions, including IA. The few existing publications on the treatment for IA primarily involved cognitive–behavioral therapy (CBT) (Du et al., 2010; Fang-ru and Wei, 2005; Kim et al., 2012; Rong et al., 2005; Young, 2007), motivational interviewing (MI) (Orzack et al., 2006; Shek et al., 2009), reality therapy (Kim, 2008), and group therapy (Cao et al., 2007; Du et al., 2010; Kim, 2008; Orzack et al., 2006; Shek et al., 2009; Zhong et al., 2009).

Two studies employed randomized designs. Du et al. (2010) randomized 56 adolescents to a no treatment control condition or an eight-session multimodal school-based group involving MI and CBT. Internet use, time management, and emotional, cognitive, and behavioral indices were assessed at baseline, post-treatment, and at a 6-month follow-up. Participants assigned to both conditions decreased Internet use to a similar degree, but those assigned to the multimodal group demonstrated improved time management skills and reductions in emotional, cognitive, and behavioral symptoms. Su et al. (2011) developed a computerized intervention that integrates MI and CBT techniques to assist college students with IA. In total, 65 students were randomly assigned to one of four conditions: the online system within a laboratory environment, the online system in their own natural environment, a non-interactive system that involved the same content as the online program but without tailored feedback, or no-treatment control. Participants were assessed pre-randomization and 1 month later. Participants in all three active treatment conditions evidenced similar reductions in hours spent online and symptoms of IA relative to those in the no-treatment control condition, suggesting potential effectiveness of this approach to treating IA. However, the sample sizes were small, the follow-up period was short, and both studies involved no-treatment control conditions, which may influence expectancy effects.

Given the paucity of randomized controlled studies, we next describe a treatment approach for IA that involves a similar, but more intensive and comprehensive, approach as those outlined previously. In particular, we focus on methods used at the Addiction Medicine Center, General

Hospital of Beijing Military Region, which has treated by far the greatest number of persons with IA in the world.

The Addiction Medicine Center in General Hospital of Beijing Military Region was founded in March 2005. It provides treatment for all types of adolescent psychological illnesses, especially IA. During approximately the past 10 years, 6,000 inpatients with IA have been treated, most of whom were males aged 15 to 19 years. Typically, the course of treatment is 3 months. A 1-year follow-up study was conducted in July 2008. Of 306 patients who completed this treatment and whose parents could be followed up by telephone or interview, a "good" or "moderate" response was found in 76.8% of the sample. The treatment approach is outlined next.

Psychotherapy

Our treatment is mainly based on CBT and Relationship Development Intervention (RDI). The goal of CBT is to teach patients to distinguish cognitions or thoughts that lead to, and stem from, problematic behaviors such as excessive Internet use; it also assists patients to identify maladaptive cognitions and apply alternative and healthier behaviors for managing them. The goal of RDI is to better connect internal moods with interpersonal relationships. Through improved interpersonal relationships, individuals can develop more positive interpersonal styles and better manage unhealthy emotions. Both approaches are premised on the clinical impression that these youth use the Internet to cope with or avoid negative emotions.

Treatment of IA generally flows through the following phases:

1. Adapting to the environment without the Internet
2. Establishing consultant–visitor relationships
3. Stimulating motivation to seek help
4. Presenting and exploring problems
5. Self-revealing and self-reflecting

6. Releasing emotions and departing from the past

7. Reconstructing adaptive cognitions and behaviors

8. Examining new cognitions and behaviors

9. Consolidating therapeutic outcomes

10. Returning to reality

The psychotherapy in our center includes group therapy, individual therapy, and family therapy.

GROUP THERAPY

Group therapy is the primary therapeutic mode. It is applied to both the patients and their parents. The patients groups are composed of patients with similar age and educational levels, and the parent groups involve parents of children of similar ages and education. The groups are intended to motivate individuals to observe, learn, and apply new information and attitudes through interpersonal interactions.

Because these patients commonly have unhealthy interpersonal relationships (parent–child, teacher–student, and friendship), group therapy encourages positive interpersonal connections and secure, stable, and warm atmospheres. Game and art therapies are applied to help patients explore and identify problematic thoughts and behaviors. Group leaders guide patients to identify their own and their peers' potential as well as shortcomings, with the goal of catalyzing positive change. Through the interpersonal group interactions, patients receive clear and comprehensive feedback regarding their interpersonal communication patterns from peers and group leaders. Group leaders apply CBT approaches to change self-cognitions, improve self-awareness, and establish new behaviors and cognitions. At the same time, the group leaders design group activities to foster positive interpersonal communications and relationships. The goal is for patients to identify unhealthy cognitions and interpersonal interactions, gain self-respect and self-confidence, and motivate self-change.

The family environment plays a role in the development of IA, and to reduce problems with IA, the home environment must also change.

Therefore, it is critical to involve parents in the treatment process. In our experience, the mothers of patients with IA have obsessive–compulsive tendencies, anxiety and depression, and employ manipulative parenting practices. The fathers often appear to be workaholics, and substance abuse is common. Their parenting style tends to include aspects of spoiling with respect to material goods but neglecting in emotional interactions. They usually believe that the IA of their child has nothing to do with them or their parenting, and they often avoid participating actively in the group therapy. With attitudes of "entrusting their children to the center," they tend to avoid therapy for themselves. To circumvent failures to participate, we require every parent to attend the lectures and parent groups from the initiation of treatment.

The parent group starts by establishing connections and developing an environment of mutual help. The parents who have been involved in treatment for longer periods are entrusted to help the newcomers by sharing experiences. Through interacting with other parents, they can identify parenting styles, couple relationships, and maladaptive cognitive processes. Group leaders direct and intervene as needed to assist parents in reducing feelings of guilt or failure and improving bonding with their children. Goals are to improve parenting style and couple relationships while better understanding their own emotions and the roles they play in their child's IA. Supportive therapy, cognitive therapy, relaxation therapy, behavior training, psychodrama (role playing), family psychotherapy, solution-focused brief therapy, transactional analysis, and Gestalt psychotherapy are used in the group session. Thus, we apply a highly comprehensive mode of psychological intervention.

INDIVIDUAL THERAPY

The treatment also involves individual therapy, in which the therapists sympathize with the patients, explore their negative feelings and prior histories of trauma, and help patients participate more fully in group therapy. Techniques include CBT, psychoanalytic, humanistic, and motivational therapy, with different emphasis depending on the primary presenting problems of the patient.

Family Therapy

Peukert et al. (2010) suggested that interventions with family members and other relatives could be useful. The families of our patients tend to be troubled with unhealthy parent–child and couples relationships, a reluctance of parents to listen to their child, perceptions of the child related to the absence of paternal love, and manipulative and irresponsible parenting styles. In the early phase of family therapy, these adverse interactions and parenting styles can emerge, providing important information for the next stage of treatment. In the intermediate phase, the therapist helps the parents use what they learned in group and family therapy to encourage their child to express and release emotions. In the mid- to late phase, all family members are encouraged to express their feelings and inner desires and to discuss solutions among all family members. The later stage of family therapy focuses on developing a specific target and plan to achieve the desired outcome.

Pharmacotherapy

As reviewed previously, IA shares some similarities with other behavioral addictions and substance use disorders (Liu et al., 2010), and the vast majority—up to 86% (Block, 2008)—of persons with IA have a comorbid psychiatric diagnosis. In our center, the three most common types of psychiatric conditions that occur with IA are ADHD, anxiety disorders, and mood disorders. Pharmacotherapy of comorbid psychiatric symptoms or disorders is important to optimize outcomes of IA (Huang et al., 2010). Reports exist regarding the use of bupropion (Han and Renshaw, 2012; Han et al., 2012), naltrexone (Bostwick and Bucci, 2008), escitalopram (Dell'Osso et al., 2008), and methylphenidate (Han et al., 2009) in treating IA and its concomitant symptoms. We regularly provide pharmacotherapies for these co-occurring disorders, along with psychotherapy.

Education

In family therapy for adolescents with IA, Young (2009) believes that educating the whole family is critical. Family members are taught methods for managing anger, handling distrust, and minimizing triggers for relapse. In addition, education, in the format of lectures and in the context of individual, family, and group therapy, is provided to address physical and mental development of the adolescents. These lectures include topics of recovery, meanings of life, personality development, and ideas of love and marriage. Successful graduates of the program are invited to return to the center to share with others their experiences and also their feelings and accomplishments following treatment. This can have a powerful effect on current patients.

BEHAVIOR TRAINING

In our center, most patients with IA lack social skills and abilities to live independently and responsibly. Behavior training is provided to cultivate appropriate behaviors and habits, self-discipline, and time management. Participation in sports is encouraged to improve health and reduce anxiety and depression.

SOCIAL EXPERIENCE

Because of poor social and communication skills, we also provide various social activities to IA patients. Our center organizes visits to orphanages and retirement communities, and it encourages participation in work programs. Through these social experiences, patients can see other perspectives and provide assistance to disadvantaged groups. The aim is to enhance gratitude for their own living environments and parents and improve their appreciation of their own situations.

Through this comprehensive and multidisciplinary approach, we have experienced success in reducing IA. However, this approach is residential and long term, typically lasting 3 months. It is in many ways culturally tailored, although many aspects appear similar to those provided to individuals with IA in Western countries. Although the treatment described here is widely applied in China, its efficacy has not been evaluated in the context of a randomized controlled trial. Thus, additional research must be undertaken before it can be considered an empirically based approach toward treating IA. Moreover, it is primarily applied with adolescents, and modifications are likely needed for treating adults with IA.

FUTURE DIRECTIONS

Although the current state of research suggests that IA may exist as a psychiatric disorder, a number of questions remain. The main issue is to establish whether this is a unique disease entity and if all aspects of problematic Internet use are best considered together under one rubric or separately. In other words, using social networks excessively may be very different from gaming excessively, which in turn may be distinct from problematic pornography viewing and Internet gaming. To this end, studies using parallel instruments are needed to compare use and problems arising from different Internet activities. The goal should be to examine differences and commonalities between various Internet applications, impairments arising from them, and persons developing problems with them, from social, functional, and biological perspectives. Another and related necessary step is to examine similarities and differences between Internet use problems that may be better explained by other disorders (e.g., online gambling as gambling disorder, online gaming as Internet gaming disorder, and types of excessive online pornography viewing as a sexual disorder). These studies will necessitate the use of large and representative samples from the general population, as well as treatment-seeking populations.

Prior to performing any such large-scale studies, however, is the need to achieve consensus on the defining features of IA and development of instruments with strong indices of reliability and validity in assessing these features. The DSM-5 criteria proposed for Internet Gaming Disorder may serve as an initial step in this direction.

Research on IA is still in its infancy, but this is an issue that has garnered international attention. Efforts to better define clinically significant harms related to excessive Internet use should be undertaken because all societies are facing a phenomenon that will persist and likely increase in the future. We need to be prepared to better understand the nature and consequences of excessive Internet use and to provide effective interventions for reducing it. In addition, development of effective prevention, and early intervention, efforts may reduce adverse public health and personal consequences of this technology.

REFERENCES

Aboujaoude, E., Koran, L.M., Gamel, N., Large, M.D., Serpe, R.T., 2006. Potential markers for problematic Internet use: A telephone survey of 2,513 adults. CNS Spectrums. 11, 750–755.

American Psychiatric Association, 2013. Diagnostic and statistical manual of mental disorders (5th ed.). Washington, DC: American Psychiatric Association.

Andreassen, C.S., Pallesen, S., 2014. Social network site addiction—An overview. Curr Pharm Design. 20, 4053–4061.

Andreassen, C.S., Torsheim, T., Brunborg, G.S., Pallesen, S., 2012. Development of a Facebook Addiction Scale. Psychol Rep. 110, 501–517.

Bakken, I.J., Wenzel, H.G., Gotestam, K.G., Johansson, A., Oren, A., 2009. Internet addiction among Norwegian adults: A stratified probability sample study. Scand J Psychol. 50, 121–127.

Block, J.J., 2008. Issues for DSM-V: Internet addiction. Am J Psychiatry. 165, 306–307.

Bostwick, J.M., Bucci, J.A., 2008. Internet sex addiction treated with naltrexone. Mayo Clin Proc. 83, 226–230.

Byun, S., Ruffini, C., Mills, J.E., Douglas, A.C., Niang, M., Stepchenkova, S., et al., 2009. Internet addiction: Metasynthesis of 1996–2006 quantitative research. Cyberpsychol Behav. 12, 203–207.

Camardese, G., De Risio, L., Di Nicola, M., Pizi, G., Janiri, L., 2012. A role for pharmacotherapy in the treatment of "Internet addiction." Clin Neuropharmacol. 35, 283–289.

Cao, F., Su, L., Gao, X., et al., 2007. Control study of group psychotherapy on middle school students with Internet overuse. Chin Ment Health J. 21, 346–358.

Carli, V., Durkee, T., Wasserman, D., Hadlaczky, G., Despalins, R., Kramarz, E., et al., 2013. The association between pathological Internet use and comorbid psychopathology: A systematic review. Psychopathology. 46, 1–13.

Chen, S.H., Weng, L.C., Su, Y.J., Wu, H.M., Yang, P.F., 2003. Development of Chinese Internet addiction scale and its psychometric study. Chin J Psychol. 45, 279–294.

Cho, S.C., Kim, J.W., Kim, B.N., Lee, J.H., Kim, E.H., 2008. Biogenetic temperament and character profiles and attention deficit hyperactivity disorder symptoms in Korean adolescents with problematic Internet use. CyberPsychol Behav. 11, 735–737.

Cox, W.M., Fadardi, J.S., Intriligator, J.M., Klinger, E., 2014. Attentional bias modification for addictive behaviors: Clinical implications. CNS Spectrums. 19, 215–224.

Davis, R.A., 2001. A cognitive–behavioral model of pathological Internet use. Computers Human Behav. 17, 187–195.

Davis, R.A., Flett, G.L., Besser, A., 2002. Validation of a new scale for measuring problematic Internet use: Implications for pre-employment screening. Cyberpsychol Behav. 5, 331–345.

Dell'Osso, B., Hadley, S., Allen, A., Baker, B., Chaplin, W.F., Hollander, E., 2008. Escitalopram in the treatment of impulsive–compulsive Internet usage disorder: An open-label trial followed by a double-blind discontinuation phase. J Clin Psychiatry. 69, 452–456.

Demetrovics, Z., Szeredi, B., Rozsa, S., 2008. The three-factor model of Internet addiction: The development of the Problematic Internet Use Questionnaire. Behav Res Methods. 40, 563–574.

Derogatis, L.R., 1975. How to use the Symptom Checklist (SCL-90) in clinical evaluations. Nutley, NY: Hofmann-La Roche.

Dong, G., Lu, Q., Zhou, H., Zhao, X., 2011. Precursor or sequela: Pathological disorders in people with Internet addiction disorder. PLoS One. 6, e14703.

Dong, G., Wang, J., Yang, X., Zhou, H., 2013. Risk personality traits of Internet addiction: A longitudinal study of Internet-addicted Chinese university students. Asia Pac Psychiatry. 5, 316–321.

Du, Y.S., Jiang, W., Vance, A., 2010. Longer term effect of randomized, controlled group cognitive behavioural therapy for Internet addiction in adolescent students in Shanghai. Aust N Z J Psychiatry. 44, 129–134.

Durkee, T., Kaess, M., Carli, V., Parzer, P., Wasserman, C., Floderus, B., et al., 2012. Prevalence of pathological Internet use among adolescents in Europe: Demographic and social factors. Addiction. 107, 2210–2222.

Fang-ru, Y., Wei, H., 2005. The effect of integrated psychosocial intervention on 52 adolescents with Internet addiction disorder. Chinese J Clin Psychol. 13(3), 343–345.

Floros, G., Siomos, K., 2013. The relationship between optimal parenting, Internet addiction and motives for social networking in adolescence. Psychiatry Res. 209, 529–534.

Gambino, B., 1997. The correction for bias in prevalence estimation with screening tests. J Gamb Stud. 13, 343–351.

Griffiths, M.D., 2005. A "components" model of addiction within a biopsychosocial framework. J Substance Use. 10, 191–197.

Guertler, D., Broda, A., Bischof, A., Kastirke, N., Meerkerk, G.J., John, U., et al., 2014a. Factor structure of the compulsive Internet use scale. Cyberpsychol Behav Soc Netw. 17, 46–51.

Guertler, D., Rumpf, H.J., Bischof, A., Kastirke, N., Petersen, K.U., John, U., et al., 2014b. Assessment of problematic Internet use by the Compulsive Internet Use Scale and the Internet Addiction Test: A sample of problematic and pathological gamblers. Eur Addict Res. 20, 75–81.

Ha, J.H., Kim, S.Y., Bae, S.C., Bae, S., Kim, H., Sim, M., et al., 2007. Depression and Internet addiction in adolescents. Psychopath. 40, 424–430.

Han, D.H., Renshaw, P.F., 2012. Bupropion in the treatment of problematic online game play in patients with major depressive disorder. J Psychopharmacol. 26, 689–696.

Han, D.H., Lee, Y.S., Na, C., Ahn, J.Y., Chung, U.S., Daniels, M.A., et al., 2009. The effect of methylphenidate on Internet video game play in children with attention-deficit/hyperactivity disorder. Compr Psychiatry. 50, 251–256.

Han, D.H., Hwang, J.W., Renshaw, P.F., 2012. Bupropion sustained release treatment decreases craving for video games and cue-induced brain activity in patients with Internet video game addiction. Exp Clin Psychopharmacol. 18, 297–304.

Huang, X.Q., Li, M.C., Tao, R., 2010. Treatment of Internet addiction. Curr Psychiatry Rep. 12, 462–470.

Huang, Z., Wang, M., Qian, M., Zhong, J., Tao, R., 2007. Chinese Internet Addiction Inventory: Developing a measure of problematic Internet use for Chinese college students. Cyberpsychol Behav. 10, 805–811.

Jelenchick, L.A., Becker, T., Moreno, M.A., 2012. Assessing the psychometric properties of the Internet Addiction Test (IAT) in U.S. college students. Psychiatry Res. 196, 296–301.

Kalaitzaki, A.E., Birtchnell, J., 2014. The impact of early parenting bonding on young adults' Internet addiction, through the mediation effects of negative relating to others and sadness. Addictive Behav. 39, 733–736.

Kim, J., 2008. The effect of a R/T group counseling program on the Internet addiction level and self-esteem of Internet addiction university students. Int J Real Ther. 27, 4–12.

Kim, S.H., Baik, S.H., Park, C.S., Kim, S.J., Choi, S.W., Kim, S.E., 2011. Reduced striatal dopamine D2 receptors in people with Internet addiction. Neuroreport. 22, 407–411.

Kim, S.M., Han, D.H., Lee, Y.S., Renshaw, P.F., 2012. Combined cognitive behavioral therapy and bupropion for the treatment of problematic on-line game play in adolescents with major depressive disorder. Comp Hum Behav. 28, 1954–1959.

Kittinger, R., Correia, C.J., Irons, J.G., 2012. Relationship between Facebook use and problematic Internet use among college students. Cyberpsychol Behav Soc Netw. 15, 324–327.

Ko, C.H., Yen, J.Y., Chen, C.S., Yeh, Y.C., Yen, C.F., 2009a. Predictive values of psychiatric symptoms for Internet addiction in adolescents: A 2-year prospective study. Arch Pediatrics Adolesc Med. 163, 937–943.

Ko, C.H., Yen, J.Y., Chen, S.H., Yang, M.J., Lin, H.C., Yen, C.F., 2009b. Proposed diagnostic criteria and the screening and diagnosing tool of Internet addiction in college students. Compr Psychiat. 50, 378–384.

Ko, C.H., Yen, J.Y., Yen, C.F., Chen, C.S., Chen, C.C., 2012. The association between Internet addiction and psychiatric disorder: A review of the literature. Eur Psychiatry. 27, 1–8.

Kuss, D.J., Griffiths, M.D., 2011. Online social networking and addiction–A review of the psychological literature. Int J Environ Res Public Health. 8, 3528–3552.

Kuss, D.J., Griffiths, M.D., Binder, J.F., 2013a. Internet addiction in students: Prevalence and risk factors. Computers Hum Behav. 29, 959–966.

Kuss, D.J., van Rooij, A.J., Shorter, G.W., Griffiths, M.D., van de Mheen, D., 2013b. Internet addiction in adolescents: Prevalence and risk factors. Comput Hum Behav. 29, 1987–1996.

Kuss, D.J., Griffiths, M.D., Karila, L., Billieux, J., 2014a. Internet addiction: A systematic review of epidemiological research for the last decade. Curr Pharm Design. 20, 4026–4052.

Kuss, D.J., Shorter, G.W., van Rooij, A.J., Griffiths, M.D., Schoenmakers, T.M., 2014b. Assessing Internet addiction using the parsimonious Internet Addiction Components Model—A preliminary study. Intern J Mental Health Addiction. 12, 351–366.

Lee, Y.S., Han, D.H., Yang, K.C., Daniels, M.A., Na, C., Kee, B.S., et al., 2008. Depression like characteristics of 5HTTLPR polymorphism and temperament in excessive Internet users. J Affect Disord. 109, 165–169.

Li, B., Friston, K.J., Liu, J., Liu, Y., Zhang, G., Cao, F., et al., 2014. Impaired frontal-basal ganglia connectivity in adolescents with Internet addiction. Sci Rep. 4, 5027.

Li, Y.J., Zhang, X.H., Lu, F.R., Zhang, Q., Wang, Y., 2014. Internet addiction among elementary and middle school students in China: A nationally representative sample study. Cyberpsychol Behav Soc Netw. 17, 111–116.

Lin, F., Zhou, Y., Du, Y., Qin, L., Zhao, Z., Xu, J., et al., 2012. Abnormal white matter integrity in adolescents with Internet addiction disorder: A tract-based spatial statistics study. PLoS One. 7, e30253.

Lin, I.H., Ko, C.H., Chang, Y.P., Liu, T.L., Wang, P.W., Lin, H.C., et al., 2014. The association between suicidality and Internet addiction and activities in Taiwanese adolescents. Comp Psychiatry. 55, 504–510.

Liu, J., Gao, X.P., Osunde, I., Li, X., Zhou, S.K., Zheng, H.R., et al., 2010. Increased regional homogeneity in Internet addiction disorder: A resting state functional magnetic resonance imaging study. Chin Med J (Engl). 123, 1904–1908.

Lortie, C.L., Guitton, M.J., 2013. Internet addiction assessment tools: Dimensional structure and methodological status. Addiction. 108, 1207–1216.

McCrae, R.R., Costa, P.T., Jr., 1987. Validation of the five-factor model of personality across instruments and observers. J Pers Soc Psychol. 52, 81–90.

Meerkerk, G.J., Van Den Eijnden, R., Vermulst, A.A., Garretsen, H.F.L., 2009. The Compulsive Internet Use Scale (CIUS): Some psychometric properties. Cyberpsychol Behav. 12, 1–6.

Moreno, M.A., Jelenchick, L., Cox, E., Young, H., Christakis, D.A., 2011. Problematic Internet use among U.S. youth: A systematic review. Arch Pediatr Adolesc Med. 165, 797–805.

Müller, K.W., Koch, A., Dickenhorst, U., Beutel, M.E., Duven, E., Wölfling, K., 2013. Addressing the question of disorder-specific risk factors of Internet addiction: A comparison of personality traits in patients with addictive behaviors and comorbid Internet addiction. Biomed Res Int. 2013, 546342.

Müller, K.W., Glaesmer, H., Brähler, E., Wölfling, K., Beutel, M.E., 2014. Prevalence of Internet addiction in the general population: Results from a German population-based survey. Behav Information Technnol. 33(7), 757–766.

Orzack, M.H., Voluse, A.C., Wolf, D., Hennen, J., 2006. An ongoing study of group treatment for men involved in problematic Internet-enabled sexual behavior. CyberPsychol Behav. 9, 348–360.

Petry, N.M., Blanco, C., Auriacombe, M., Borges, G., Bucholz, K., Crowley, T.J., et al., 2014. An overview of and rationale for changes proposed for pathological gambling in DSM-5. J Gamb Stud. 14, 493–502.

Peukert, P., Sieslack, S., Barth, G., Batra, A., 2010. Internet and computer game addiction: Phenomenology, comorbidity, etiology, diagnostics, and therapeutic implications for the addictives and their relatives. Psychiatr Prax. 37, 219–224.

Rehbein, F., Mößle, T., 2013. Video game and Internet addiction: Is there a need for differentiation? Sucht. 59, 129–142.

Rong, Y., Zhi, S., Yong, Z., 2005. Comprehensive intervention on Internet addiction of middle school students. Chin Ment Health J. 19, 457–459.

Rumpf, H.J., Bischof, G., Bischof, A., Besser, B., Glorius, S., deBrito, S., et al., 2014a. Applying DSM-5 criteria for Internet Gaming Disorder to different Internet activities. Manuscript draft, University of Lübeck, Lübeck, Germany.

Rumpf, H.J., Vermulst, A.A., Bischof, A., Kastirke, N., Gürtler, N., Bischof, G., et al., 2014b. Occurence of Internet addiction in a general population sample: A latent class analysis. Eur Addiction Res. 20, 159–166.

Sariyska, R., Reuter, M., Bey, K., Sha, P., Li, M., Chen, Y.F., et al., 2014. Self-esteem, personality and Internet addiction: A cross-cultural comparison study. Pers Individ Differ. 61/62, 28–33.

Servidio, R., 2014. Exploring the effects of demographic factors, Internet usage and personality traits on Internet addiction in a sample of Italian university students. Computers Hum Behav. 35, 85–92.

Shaffer, H.J., Hall, M.N., Vander Bilt, J., 2000. "Computer addiction": A critical consideration. Am J Orthopsychiatry. 70, 162–168.

Shaw, M., Black, D.W., 2008. Internet addiction: Definition, assessment, epidemiology and clinical management. CNS Drugs. 22, 353–365.

Shek, D.T., Tang, V.M., Lo, C.Y., 2009. Evaluation of an Internet addiction treatment program for Chinese adolescents in Hong Kong. Adolescence. 44, 359–373.

Sim, T., Gentile, D.A., Bricolo, F., Serpelloni, G., Gulamoydeen, F., 2012. A conceptual review of research on the pathological use of computers, video games, and the Internet. Int J Mental Health Addiction. 10, 748–769.

Siomos, K., Floros, G., Fisoun, V., Evaggelia, D., Farkonas, N., Sergentani, E., et al., 2012. Evolution of Internet addiction in Greek adolescent students over a two-year period: The impact of parental bonding. Eur Child Adolescent Psychiatry. 21, 211–219.

Steffen, S., Peukert, P., Petersen, K.U., Batra, A., 2012. Messverfahren zur Erfassung der Internetsucht. Sucht. 58, 401–413.

Su, W., Fang, X., Miller, J.K., Wang, Y., 2011. Internet-based intervention for the treatment of online addiction for college students in China: A pilot study of the Healthy Online Self-Helping Center. Cyberpsychol Behav Soc Netw. 14, 497–503.

Tao, R., Huang, X.Q., Wang, J.N., Zhang, H.M., Zhang, Y., Li, M.C., 2010. Proposed diagnostic criteria for Internet addiction. Addiction. 105, 556–564.

Tsai, H.F., Cheng, S.H., Yeh, T.L., Shih, C.C., Chen, K.C., Yang, Y.C., et al., 2009. The risk factors of Internet addiction—A survey of university freshmen. Psychiatry Res. 167, 294–299.

van der Aa, N., Overbeek, G., Engels, R.C., Scholte, R.H., Meerkerk, G.J., Van den Eijnden, R.J., 2009. Daily and compulsive Internet use and well-being in adolescence: A diathesis-stress model based on big five personality traits. J Youth Adolesc. 38, 765–776.

Volkow, N.D., Fowler, J.S., Wang, G.J., 2004. The addicted human brain viewed in the light of imaging studies: Brain circuits and treatment strategies. Neuropharmacology. 47(Suppl 1), 3–13.

Widyanto, L., McMurran, M., 2004. The psychometric properties of the Internet Addiction Test. CyberPsychol Behav. 7, 443–450.

Wurst, F.M., Rumpf, H.J., Skipper, G.E., Allen, J.P., Kunz, I., Beschoner, P., et al., 2013. Estimating the prevalence of drinking problems among physicians. Gen Hosp Psychiatry. 35, 561–564.

Xiuqin, H., Huimin, Z., Mengchen, L., Jinan, W., Ying, Z., Ran, T., 2010. Mental health, personality, and parental rearing styles of adolescents with Internet addiction disorder. Cyberpsychol Behav Soc Netw. 13, 401–406.

Xu, J., Shen, L.X., Yan, C.H., Hu, H., Yang, F., Wang, L., et al., 2014. Parent–adolescent interaction and risk of adolescent Internet addiction: A population-based study in Shanghai. BMC Psychiatry. 14, 112.

Yao, M.Z., He, J., Ko, D.M., Pang, K.C., 2014. The influence of personality, parental behaviors, and self-esteem on Internet addiction: A study of Chinese college students. Cyberpsychol Behav Soc Netw. 17, 104–110.

Young, K., 2009. Understanding online gaming addiction and treatment issues for adolescents. Am J Ther. 37, 355–372.

Young, K.S., 1998a. Caught in the net: How to recognize the signs of Internet addiction—and a winning strategy for recovery. New York: Wiley.

Young, K.S., 1998b. Internet addiction: The emergence of a new clinical disorder. Cyberpsychol Behav. 1, 237–244.

Young, K.S., 2007. Treatment outcomes using CBT-IA with Internet-addicted patients. J Behav Addict. 2, 209–215.

Young, K.S., Pistner, M., O'Mara, J., Buchanan, J., 1999. Cyber disorders: The mental health concern for the new millennium. CyberPsychol Behav. 2, 475–479.

Yuan, K., Qin, W., Wang, G., Zeng, F., Zhao, L., Yang, X., et al., 2011. Microstructure abnormalities in adolescents with Internet addiction disorder. PLoS One. 6, e20708.

Zhang, H.X., Jiang, W.Q., Lin, Z.G., Du, Y.S., Vance, A., 2013. Comparison of psychological symptoms and serum levels of neurotransmitters in Shanghai adolescents with and without Internet addiction disorder: A case–control study. PLoS One. 8, 4.

Zhang, J., Xin, T., 2013. Measurement of Internet addiction: An item response analysis approach. Cyberpsychol Behav Soc Netw. 16, 464–468.

Zhong, X., Tao, R., Zu, S., et al., 2009. Effect of group psychological intervention in adolescents on Internet addiction. J Capital Med Univ. 30, 494–499.

Zhou, Y., Lin, F.C., Du, Y.S., Qin, L.D., Zhao, Z.M., Xu, J.R., et al., 2011. Gray matter abnormalities in Internet addiction: A voxel-based morphometry study. Eur J Radiol. 79, 92–95.

5

Hypersexual Disorder

MEGAN M. CAMPBELL AND DAN J. STEIN ■

Clinicians have long been aware of patients with symptoms of hypersexual disorder, also referred to in the literature as sexual addiction, compulsive sexual behavior, impulsive–compulsive sexual behavior, hyperphilia, and paraphilia-related disorder. This chapter provides an overview of the literature on hypersexual disorder, including recently proposed diagnostic criteria for the fifth edition of the *Diagnostic and statistical manual of mental disorders* (DSM-5; American Psychiatric Association, 2013). Different models used to conceptualize the disorder are discussed in terms of phenomenology, psychobiology, and assessment. These include a sexual desire dysregulation model; a sexual addiction and dependency model; sexual compulsivity models; and an ABC model of affective dysregulation (A), behavioral addiction (B), and cognitive dyscontrol (C). The chapter presents available information on prevalence rates of hypersexual disorder, and it describes comorbidities between hypersexual disorder and other psychiatric conditions, including substance use disorders, anxiety disorders, mood disorders, impulse control disorders, and personality disorders. Demographic, neurophysiological, genetic, and family risk factors are outlined. Psychopharmacology and psychotherapy treatment options are discussed, and future research directions are suggested.

DEFINING FEATURES AND METHODS FOR ASSESSMENT

Clinical accounts of excessive, maladaptive sexual behavior including compulsive masturbation have been reported as early as the 18th century, whereas terms such as Don Juanism, satyriasis, and nymphomania were used in the 19th century to refer to male and female promiscuity (Kafka, 2010). In the following sections, we discuss the classification of such behavior in contemporary nosological systems and also more recent theoretical approaches to its conceptualization.

Current Psychiatric Classification Systems

Within the DSM, distress as a result of sexual behavior was first proposed in the DSM-III, under the diagnostic category "Psychosexual Disorder Not Otherwise Specified" (American Psychiatric Association, 1980). This referred to "distress about a pattern of repeated sexual conquests with a succession of individuals who exist only as things to be used" (American Psychiatric Association, 1980. p. 283). This category was revised in the DSM-III-R to include the concept of non-paraphilic sexual addiction and renamed "Sexual Disorders Not Otherwise Specified" (American Psychiatric Association, 1986). However, due to a lack of empirical evidence, sexual addiction was removed from the DSM-IV and DSM-IV-TR, and the DSM-III diagnostic criteria for "Psychosexual Disorder Not Otherwise Specified" were re-established (Kafka, 2010).

During the DSM-5 revision process, hypersexual disorder was proposed as a new diagnostic category (Kafka, 2010). The DSM-5 Sexual Disorders Workgroup defined hypersexual disorder as a "sexual desire disorder characterized by an increased frequency and intensity of sexually motivated fantasies, arousal, urges, and enacted behavior in association with an impulsivity component—a maladaptive behavioral response with adverse consequences" resulting in clinically significant personal distress or social, occupational, or other impairment and not due to the physiological effect of an exogenous substance (e.g., drug of abuse or medication) (Kafka, 2010, p. 385).

Initially proposed diagnostic criteria included at least three of the following experienced over a 6-month period (Kafka, 2010):

1. Time consumed by sexual fantasies, urges, or behaviors that repetitively interfere with other important (nonsexual) goals, activities, and obligations
2. Repetitive engaging in sexual fantasies, urges, or behaviors in response to dysphoric mood states (e.g., anxiety, depression, boredom, and irritability)
3. Repetitive engaging in sexual fantasies, urges, or behaviors in response to stressful life events
4. Repetitive but unsuccessful efforts to control or significantly reduce these sexual fantasies, urges, or behaviors
5. Repetitive engaging in these sexual behaviors while disregarding the risk for physical or emotional harm to self or others

Proposed specifiers included excessive masturbation, pornography use, sexual behavior with consenting adults, cybersex, telephone sex, strip clubs, and other.

A DSM-5 field trial evaluated the reliability, validity, and clinical utility of the proposed hypersexual disorder diagnostic criteria in a sample of 207 outpatients seeking treatment for hypersexual disorder, substance use disorders, or general psychiatric conditions (Reid et al., 2012). The study used structured diagnostic interviews and self-report inventories. Findings demonstrated good internal consistency and good stability over time for these proposed criteria. The criteria demonstrated validity in comparison with theoretically related measures of stress, impulsivity, and emotional dysregulation, and sensitivity and specificity indicators suggested that the criteria accurately reflected the disorder among the patients sampled. Masturbation, pornography use, and sexual behavior with consenting adults were the most commonly endorsed specifiers.

These results provided evidence of the reliability and validity of diagnostic criteria for a condition characterized by intense, dysregulated preoccupation with sexual fantasies and behaviors, leading to adverse consequences and impairment in social and occupational functioning. However, the question of whether such a condition is a distinct entity with clinical significance remained controversial (Hartmann, 2013). Because there is no consistent, normative pattern of sexual behavior cross-culturally, a diagnosis of hypersexual disorder arguably also holds the risk of labeling adaptive human behavior as a mental disorder (Kaplan and Krueger, 2010). Furthermore, hypersexual behavior demonstrates high comorbidity with other psychiatric and medical conditions, and critics have suggested hypersexual behavior is merely indicative of another underlying mental disorder (Kaplan and Krueger, 2010).

Although hypersexual disorder was ultimately rejected for inclusion in the DSM-5 due to limited empirical evidence related to etiology, prevalence, and treatment, as well as a lack of expert consensus on how to conceptualize the disorder (Hartmann, 2013), compulsive sexual disorder, another term used in the literature to describe hypersexual disorder, is being considered for inclusion as one of the impulse control disorders in the International Statistical Classification of Diseases and Related Health Problems, version 11 (ICD-11; Grant et al., 2014). The ICD-10 currently includes the diagnoses of "excessive masturbation" and "excessive sexual drive" with a subdivision of "satyriasis" for men and "nymphomania" for women (World Health Organization, 2007). However, these terms have been criticized for their focus on excessive sexual behavior, which remains undefined (Kor et al., 2013) and holds the risk of pathologizing normative patterns of sexual behavior (Kaplan and Krueger, 2010).

In summary, the diagnosis of hypersexual disorder is not currently included in the DSM or the ICD, but compulsive sexuality is currently being considered for inclusion in the ICD-11. If agreement is achieved regarding the inclusion of this diagnosis in a major diagnostic manual, it will pave the way for additional research on the etiology and treatment of the condition. The DSM-5 did not include the disorder in part due to a lack of expert consensus on models for conceptualizing the disorder. In the following section, dominant models of conceptualizing hypersexual disorder are discussed.

Models of Hypersexual Disorder and Methods of Assessment

Different models have been proposed for conceptualizing hypersexual disorder, including the sexual desire dysregulation model (Kafka, 2010); a sexual addiction and dependency model (Kor et al., 2013; Rosenberg et al., 2013); sexual compulsivity and impulsivity models (Kuzma and Black, 2008); and an ABC model of affective dysregulation (A), behavioral addiction (B), and cognitive dyscontrol (C) that includes both impulsive and compulsive features (Stein, 2008). We discuss each in turn, describing possible theories of phenomenology, psychobiology, and assessment.

Sexual Desire Dysregulation Model

Sexual desire is defined as the sexual fantasies, urges, or activities that consciously motivate engagement in sexual behaviors in response to internal or external stimuli (Kafka, 2010). Hypersexual disorder may be conceptualized as resulting from sexual desire dysregulation, with increased frequency and intensity in sexually motivated fantasies (Kafka, 2010).

One approach has defined sexual desire dysregulation solely in terms of behavior. Frequency of sexual behavior has been quantified using the term total sexual outlet (TSO) per week (Kinsey et al., 1948). This measure accounts for the total number of orgasms achieved by an individual through any single or combined sexual behavior (including masturbation, sexual intercourse, and/or oral sex). Kafka (1997) initially proposed that a TSO of 7 per week be used as a diagnostic indicator of hypersexual disorder. However, such a proposal runs the risk of pathologizing normative sexual behavior that did not cause distress or dysfunction or the potential problem of not recognizing pathological sexual behavior that did not culminate in orgasm (Kingston and Firestone, 2008).

Another variation of the sexual desire dysregulation model has hypothesized a central set of opposing neurobiological processes, responsible for sexual activation/excitation and sexual inhibition (Bancroft et al., 2009). Although degrees of sexual excitation and inhibition vary across

individuals, sexual behavior remains largely adaptive and nonproblem-
atic. However, unusually high sexual activation or excitation and low
inhibition may result in high-risk, problematic sexual behavior, whereas
low sexual activation or excitation and high inhibition may result in
problems in sexual response or sexual dysfunction (Bancroft et al., 2009).
It has been hypothesized that enhanced dopaminergic neurotransmission is associated with sexual excitation, whereas enhanced serotonergic
neurotransmission is associated with sexual inhibition (Kafka, 2010).
However, to date, no sensitive or specific biomarkers of sexual dysregulation are available, and this model remains speculative.

Assessment tools such as the Sexual Excitation Scale (SES) and Sexual
Inhibition Scales (SIS1 and SS2) (Janssen et al., 2002a, 2002b) have been
developed based on the dual control model of sexual arousal (Bancroft
et al., 2009). The SES and SIS have been used to assess sexual arousal,
sexual appetite, and sexual risk-taking. Findings suggest a relationship
between high sexual arousal/excitation, low inhibition, and increased
sexual promiscuity and masturbation, particularly in individuals with
anxiety and depressive symptoms (Kafka, 2010).

The Hypersexual Behavior Inventory (HBI) (Reid et al., 2011) draws
heavily from the criteria proposed for DSM-5 and includes features of
this sexual desire dysregulation model. This inventory has 19 items
that are rated on a 5-point scale, with scores of 53 out of 95 considered to reflect diagnosis. The scale has three subscales: (1) control over
sexual thoughts, urges, and behavior; (2) consequences associated
with hypersexual behavior; and (3) extent to which sex is used to cope
with uncomfortable or unpleasant affective experiences (Marshall and
Briken, 2010). Scores on the HBI correlate with impaired executive
functioning and specifically with disturbed emotional self-regulation,
problem-solving, planning, and self-management (Marshall and
Briken, 2010).

Whereas the sexual desire dysregulation model proposes a focus on the
association between negative affect and increased frequency and intensity
of sexually motivated fantasies and behavior, a different model of hypersexual disorder is based on behavioral addiction.

SEXUAL ADDICTION AND SEXUAL DEPENDENCE MODEL

Behavioral addictions are characterized by several core elements, including salience (the behavior dominates the person's thinking, feelings, and behaviors), mood modification (emotional effect of the behavior and its use as a coping mechanism), tolerance (increasing amounts of the behavior are needed to achieve the same emotional effect), withdrawal symptoms (unpleasant feeling states and physical effects resulting from not engaging in the behavior), conflict (intrapsychic, interpersonal, work, and social resulting from engaging in the behavior), and relapse (tendency to return to extreme patterns of the addictive behavior) (Rosenberg and Curtis Feder, 2014). These may be applied to a range of behaviors, including sex.

A behavioral addiction model of sexual behavior may emphasize the role of reward circuitry. Evidence suggests that sexual arousal and orgasm are mediated by the mesolimbic reward system including the striatum, medial prefrontal cortex, and orbitofrontal cortex (Kor et al., 2013). Neural circuitry connecting the ventral tegmental area and nucleus accumbens regulates reward processes in the brain, and the dopaminergic neurotransmitter system plays a key role in these pathways (Rosenberg et al., 2013). The model hypothesizes that this circuitry plays an important role in mediating sexual addiction (Rosenberg et al., 2013).

Conceptualizing hypersexual disorder as a sexual addiction leads to an emphasis on particular constructs when assessing patients. It suggests the repetitive, maladaptive use of sexual behaviors to manage negative effects, with increased tolerance and risk-taking over time, a loss of control over the behavior coupled with adverse psychosocial consequences, and the experience of withdrawal when the behavior is stopped (Carnes, 1983). Motivation–reward, affect regulation, and behavior inhibition are key considerations in assessment (Goodman, 2008).

Although sexual addiction is not currently included in the DSM-5, it has contributed toward strengthening the construct of behavior addictions, and "Internet Gaming Disorder" has been added to Section 3 of the DSM-5 as a provisional "behavior addiction" worthy of further research (Rosenberg et al., 2014). Instruments such as the 25-item Sexual

Addictions Screening Test (SAST) (Carnes, 1989) have been developed as screening tools for sexual addiction. The SAST has demonstrated good internal consistency, construct validity, and factor structure as a measure of sexual addiction (Marshall and Briken, 2010).

Whereas the sexual addiction and sexual dependence model focuses on hypersexual disorder as a behavioral addiction with motivation–reward, affect regulation, and behavior inhibition as key considerations, a third model emphasizes sexual compulsivity.

SEXUAL COMPULSIVITY AND SEXUAL IMPULSIVITY MODELS

Conceptualizing hypersexual disorder as an obsessive–compulsive and related disorder suggests the repetitive use of sexual behaviors to reduce anxiety and other negative effects (Kafka, 2010). This model overlaps considerably with the sexual desire dysregulation model, but it emphasizes obsessive–compulsive features: Sexual obsessions in the form of increasingly time-consuming sexual fantasies may be used ritualistically to distract from and negate negative emotions (Kor et al., 2013).

Sexual compulsivity is associated with volitional impairment and sexual sensation-seeking and risk-taking behavior, intrinsically driven by anxiety (Kafka, 2010; Kuzma and Black, 2008). However, hypersexual disorder is characterized by pleasure-seeking behavior, suggesting the involvement of reward circuitry. Sexual risk-taking and sexual sensation-seeking behaviors overlap with sexual impulsivity (Kafka, 2010). As a result, sexual impulsivity may be a preferred model of pathophysiology because of the intrinsically enjoyable nature of sex aligning with the pleasure-seeking motivations of impulsivity (Giugliano, 2013).

The Sexual Compulsivity Scale (SCS), the Sexual Sensation Seeking Scale (SSSS) (Kalichman and Rompa, 1995; Kalichman et al., 1994), and the Compulsive Sexual Behavior Inventory (CSBI) (Coleman et al., 2001) have been developed to assess sexual compulsion and sexual risk-taking behavior (Kafka, 2010). The SCS and CSBI have demonstrated correlations between hypersexual behavior and engaging in high-risk sex and tendencies toward sexual coercion, poor emotional self-regulation, poor relationship intimacy, and low sexual contentment (Marshall and Briken, 2010).

Arguably, hypersexual disorder shares both compulsive and impulsive features. Whereas pleasure and arousal may be associated with impulsive features that initiate the disorder, more compulsive components may maintain the behavior over time (Kor et al., 2013). Alternatively, some individuals may engage in hypersexual behavior to manage and alleviate negative affective states suggesting more compulsive tendencies (Kingston and Firestone, 2008). Such patients may report feelings of guilt and regret following these compulsive sexual behaviors. Other individuals may engage in hypersexual behavior to enhance positive emotional states, a pattern suggesting more impulsive tendencies (Kingston and Firestone, 2008). Such patients may demonstrate an inability to delay sexual gratification and impulsive decision-making.

An ABC Model of Affective Dysregulation (A), Behavioral Addiction (B), and Cognitive Dyscontrol (C)

When conceptualizing hypersexual disorder as an impulse control problem, an ABC model of affective dysregulation (A), behavioral addiction (B), and cognitive dyscontrol (C) may be useful. This model integrates some features of the sexual desire dysregulation model, the sexual addiction and sexual dependence model, and the sexual compulsivity and impulsivity models (Stein, 2008).

Hypersexual behavior may be triggered as a result of stress and negative affect, suggesting a degree of affect dysregulation (A) (Stein, 2008). The psychobiology of stress-induced impulsivity suggests that amygdala activation may play a particularly important role. In addition, many patients with hypersexual disorder have comorbid mood and anxiety disorders, providing further support for the association between affect dysregulation and symptoms of the disorder.

Behavioral addictive (B) features of hypersexual behavior are demonstrated in the individual's preoccupation with his or her sexual desires that gradually increase in frequency and intensity, consistent with tolerance, and cause dysphoria when discontinued (Stein, 2008). Ventral striatal circuitry, and the nucleus accumbens in particular, may play an important role here. The ability of behaviors to regulate emotions has been a primary argument for including behavior addictions in the addiction model (Kingston and Firestone, 2008).

Inability to fully process cognitively or affectively the medium- and long-term consequences of these sexual impulses suggests a degree of cognitive dyscontrol (C) (Stein, 2008). Cognitive dyscontrol may be further demonstrated at a neuropsychological level through impaired executive control on systematic testing and at a biological level through decreased prefrontal activation (Stein, 2008).

An ABC model attempts to integrate the affective dysregulation prominent in the sexual desire dysregulation and compulsive sexuality models, with features of the behavioral addiction model, and cognitive dyscontrol central to the impulsive sexuality model. This integrative approach promotes investigation of different phenomenological and psychobiological components of hypersexual disorder instead of relying on a single theoretical approach. It raises the question of whether dimensions of symptoms are underpinned by different brain regions and whether these shed light on underlying biology as well as on clinical treatment.

PREVALENCE RATES

No large-scale epidemiological studies of hypersexual disorder have been conducted, partly due to the lack of consensus about how to conceptualize and define hypersexual disorder and how to measure it (Marshall and Briken, 2010). Prevalence of sexual addiction has been estimated at between 3% and 6% of the general U.S. adult population (Carnes, 1991; Kuzma and Black, 2008), although methods and criteria for establishing these estimates remain undecided (Marshall and Briken, 2010). Higher rates have been reported in one sexual offender population study; using the SAST, Marshall and Marshall (2006) reported prevalence rates of 40% in a sample of 40 U.S. sexual offenders in comparison with 17% in a community comparison group.

Data on frequency of orgasm in terms of TSO per week have been used to identify a population characterized by increased frequency of sexual behavior (Kafka, 2010). A U.S. sexuality survey of 1,320 men aged between 18 and 59 years reported that only 1.9% masturbated daily, and only 7.6% engaged in sexual intercourse with their partners four or more times per week (Laumann et al., 1994). Similarly, a Swedish general population survey ($N = 2,450$) indicated that only 12.1% of men reported four or more orgasms per week, and only 6.8% of women reported three or more orgasms per week (Långström and Hanson, 2006). In comparison, within a sample of U.S. men receiving treatment for paraphilia-related conditions, 90% reported five or more orgasms per week (Kafka, 1997).

Research suggests that within this population, there is a subgroup in which increased frequency and intensity of sexual behavior leads to distress and impairment in life functioning (Kafka, 2010). Within this subgroup, hypersexual behavior is associated with increased risk-taking behavior and sexually transmitted infections (STIs), dissatisfaction in sexual relationships, interpersonal difficulties, and increased accessing of professional services for sexuality-related problems (Långström and Hanson, 2006). Additional adverse consequences include interpersonal and relationship problems (e.g., separation and divorce), excessive financial expenses, and work and education impairments (Kafka, 2010).

COMORBIDITIES

Although the prevalence rate of hypersexual disorder is not well understood, data from treatment-seeking samples suggest that it is highly associated with other psychiatric conditions. The following sections describe the limited research on comorbidities of other mental health conditions with hypersexual disorder.

Axis I Disorders

Data from clinical samples suggest a strong association between hypersexual disorder and substance use disorders, anxiety disorders, mood disorders, and impulse control disorders (Kafka, 2010). For example, within a sample of 36 individuals with compulsive sexual behavior, 64% reported a history of substance use disorders, 50% reported a history of anxiety disorders, 39% reported a history of major depression or dysthymia, and 14% reported a lifetime prevalence of obsessive–compulsive disorder (Black et al., 1997). In a sample of 24 individuals with sexual compulsions, 100% met the diagnostic criteria for an Axis 1 disorder within their lifetime (Raymond et al., 2003). Of these individuals, 96% reported a lifetime comorbidity of anxiety disorders, 71% substance use disorders, 71% mood disorders, and 38% impulse control disorders. In addition, 46% reported a lifetime comorbidity of sexual dysfunctions. A meta-analysis involving 19 studies of 3,783 patients identified with and receiving treatment for hypersexual behavior demonstrated a moderate positive correlation ($r = .34$) of hypersexual behavior and depressive symptoms (Schultz et al., 2014). In addition, in a Swedish sample, hypersexual behavior was associated with increased risk-taking behavior that included smoking cigarettes, increased alcohol use, use of illegal substances, and gambling (Långström and Hanson, 2006).

Hypersexual disorder shows some association with other behavior addictions, such as pathological gambling. Within Black et al.'s (1997) sample of 36 individuals with compulsive sexual behavior, 11% described themselves as pathological gamblers. In one sample of 96 pathological gamblers, 9.4% reported a lifetime history of compulsive sexual behavior (Grant and Kim, 2003), and in a sample of 225 patients with problem gambling, 19.6% evidenced compulsive sexual behavior (Grant and Steinberg, 2005).

Hypersexual behavior has shown an association with attention deficit disorders and post-traumatic stress disorder (Reid et al., 2009), as well as obsessive–compulsive and related disorders (Lochner and Stein, 2010). Sexual addiction has been associated with affect dysregulation, loneliness, low self-worth, and insecure attachment styles (Rosenberg et al., 2014).

Different models of hypersexual disorder may be used to explain patterns of comorbidity. The sexual desire dysregulation model will arguably predict higher comorbidity with mood disorders, the sexual addiction and sexual dependence model will likely predict an association with substance use disorders and other behavioral addictions, a sexual compulsivity model will arguably predict higher comorbidity with obsessive–compulsive and related disorders, and a sexual impulsivity model will predict the strongest association with impulse-control disorders. Given the limited data available, none of the theories can be supported or refuted conclusively.

There is also some debate about the association between hypersexual disorder and paraphilic disorders. Both conditions are associated with intense, repetitive sexual behaviors and sexual preoccupation that intensifies during periods of stress (Kafka, 2010). In addition, both conditions show a higher prevalence in males and onset in adolescence (Kafka, 2010). However, hypersexual disorder is understood as disinhibited or excessive in comparison to normophilic sexual behaviors, whereas paraphilic disorders are considered deviant sexual preferences and deviant forms of sexual arousal (Kafka, 2010).

Axis II (Personality) Disorders

Hypersexual disorder has been associated with cluster B (antisocial, borderline, histrionic, and narcissistic) and cluster C (avoidant, dependent, and obsessive–compulsive) personality disorders as well. For example, within a sample of 36 individuals with compulsive sexual behavior, 44% met the diagnostic criteria for an Axis II disorder, of which 29% received a cluster B diagnosis and 24% cluster C (Black et al., 1997). Similarly, within a sample of 24 individuals with sexual compulsions, 46% met the diagnostic criteria for an Axis II disorder, of which 39% met the criteria for a cluster C personality disorder and 23% cluster B (Raymond et al., 2003). Paranoid, histrionic, narcissistic, avoidant, obsessive–compulsive, and passive aggressive personality types were most commonly associated with hypersexual disorder (Kafka, 2010).

In summary, hypersexual disorder has shown association with both Axis I and Axis II disorders, specifically substance use disorders, anxiety disorders, mood disorders, and impulse control disorders. However, relatively few studies of comorbidity exist, and they comprise small numbers of primarily treatment-seeking patients, who may not be representative of the larger population of persons with hypersexual disorder.

RISK AND PROTECTIVE FACTORS

Demographic Correlates

Studies report that whereas men experience increased sexual fantasies, frequency of masturbation, tendency toward external visual sexual arousal and ease of arousal, along with more accepting attitudes toward causal sex, women's sexual motivations, arousal patterns, and behaviors tend to be more context specific, motivated by biological and emotional needs (Kafka, 2010; Kaplan and Krueger, 2010). As a result, men may be more vulnerable to hypersexual behavior than women; however, there is a current lack of research focused on women in both population-based and clinically derived samples. A male:female prevalence ratio has been estimated at 5:1 (Kafka, 2010).

The majority of self-referred patients presenting for treatment of hypersexual disorder are men (Kafka, 2010). Research suggests different behavior patterns and sexual scripts for men and women presenting with hypersexual disorder (Kafka, 2010). In men, hypersexual behavior is associated with less satisfaction with sexual experiences, more interpersonal problems, more sexually transmitted diseases, and professional help-seeking for sexuality-related problems (Långström and Hanson, 2006). In terms of sexual behaviors, men are more likely than women to have more sexual partners, engage in compulsive masturbation and paraphilias, pay for sex, and engage in anonymous sex (Kuzma and Black, 2008). Women demonstrating characteristics of hypersexual behavior are more likely than their male counterparts to report a history of sexual abuse and psychiatric care (Långström and Hanson, 2006). In terms of specific sexual behaviors, women are more likely than men to engage in fantasy sex, sadomasochism, or to use sex as a business (Kuzma and Black, 2008). Both men and women engaged in hypersexual behavior tend to exhibit other risk-taking behaviors, including substance use and gambling (Långström and Hanson, 2006).

Neurobiological Risk Factors

Medical conditions such as dementia, temporal lobe epilepsy, and Tourette's syndrome have been associated with hypersexual behavior as a result of disinhibition of the limbic system, whereas frontal lesions resulting from brain injury, stroke, and frontal lobotomy have also been linked with disinhibition and hypersexual behavior (Kaplan and Krueger, 2010). Striatal lesions have been associated with repetitive triggering of internal response patterns, whereas temporal–limbic lesions have been associated with disturbances in sexual appetite and sexual drive (Stein et al., 2000).

Substance use disorders (specifically methamphetamine and cocaine abuse) and dopamine agonist treatment for Parkinson's disease have been associated with hypersexual behavior, possibly as a result of the dopaminergic system's influence on sexual appetite and drive (Kaplan and Krueger, 2010). The neurobiology underlying a potential association between these behaviors and hypersexual behavior requires further investigation.

Genetics and Family Risk Factors

Some evidence has been presented for a possible genetic predisposition toward hypersexual behavior (Kuzma and Black, 2008). For example, within a sample of 75 couples recovering from sexual addiction, 40% reported a parent with substance dependency, 36% with sexual addiction, 33% with an eating disorder, and 7% with pathological gambling (Schneider and Schneider, 1996). Monozygotic and dizygotic twin studies suggest heritability of sexual promiscuous behavior may be as high as 33% (Zietsch et al., 2010).

Research findings suggest an association between compulsive sexual behavior and a history of childhood sexual abuse (Kuzma and Black, 2008). One survey reported compulsive sexual behavior and a history of childhood sexual abuse in 80% of the sample (Carnes and Delmonico, 1996), whereas other studies have reported an association in 31% (Black et al., 1997) and 28% (Kafka and Prentky, 1992) of samples. Although the available data suggest familial environmental and possibly genetic factors that may contribute toward hypersexual disorder, more research is necessary to delineate these risk factors.

Risk-taking and Sensation-Seeking Behaviors

Hypersexual disorder is associated with preoccupation with sexual fantasies and sexual behaviors, pornography dependency, compulsive masturbation, promiscuity, and risk-taking and sensation-seeking sexual behavior (Kafka, 2010; Kaplan and Krueger, 2010; Kuzma and Black, 2008). As a result, individuals with this disorder may have increased risk of unprotected sex, leading to STIs, HIV infection, and unwanted pregnancies. Patients also report interpersonal and relationship problems, including marital separation and divorce, as well as excessive financial expenses due to sexual activities and also work and education impairments (Kafka, 2010). Supplemental reports from family members and intimate partners may provide valuable collateral information to help assess the extent of difficulties and whether any factors contribute to the onset of the condition or manifest as a consequence of it.

TREATMENTS

Individuals typically seek treatment for hypersexual behaviors as a result of a negative experience or consequence associated with their sexual behavior, such as relationship difficulties or legal problems. Both pharmacotherapy and psychotherapy have been used to treat these patients, although empirical research related to treatment is limited.

Psychopharmacology

Selective serotonin reuptake inhibitors (SSRIs) and serotonin/norepinephrine reuptake inhibitors, which are typically used as antidepressants, appear to reduce desire, arousal, and orgasm (Kingston and Firestone, 2008). Two double-blind, placebo-controlled trials have shown a decrease in hypersexual disorder symptoms with the use of antidepressant medications clomipramine, desipramine, and citalopram. A double-blind, crossover design, preceded by a 2-week single-blind placebo period, was used to compare clomipramine and desipramine in a sample of 15 patients with paraphilias (Kruesi et al., 1992). The 8 patients who completed the trial showed a reduction in paraphilic symptoms with the use of both medications, in comparison with baseline measures. No difference in treatment affect was indicated between the two medications. In a double-blind study of citalopram versus placebo for the treatment of compulsive sexuality in a sample of 28 gay and bisexual men, citalopram demonstrated a reduction in sexual desire, sexual drive, frequency of masturbation, and pornography use (Wainberg et al., 2006). However, sexual risk-taking behavior remained unchanged. These trials provide limited initial potential for the use of antidepressant medication in the treatment of hypersexual disorder, but larger randomized controlled trials are needed to evaluate their efficacy (Marshall and Briken, 2010).

There are also case series reporting potential benefits of SSRIs, psychostimulants, and triptorelin in hypersexual disorder (Kaplan and Krueger, 2010; Marshall and Briken, 2010; Stein et al., 1992). Mood stabilizers and anti-impulsive medications have been suggested for managing patients presenting with manic or impulsive features or promiscuity, whereas stimulants have been suggested for highly distractible and thrill-seeking individuals (Kingston and Firestone, 2008). Case reports have also suggested that treatment of hypersexual disorder with naltrexone, nefazodone, and valproic acid may be useful (Kaplan and Krueger, 2010). However, no double-blind, randomized clinical trials exist to support the use of mood stabilizers or anti-impulsive medications in hypersexual disorder.

Psychotherapies

Different psychotherapy approaches have been suggested for the support and treatment of hypersexual disorder, placing emphasis on different aspects of the patient's presenting problem. As in the case of pharmacotherapies, there are few randomized control trials to demonstrate the efficacy of these approaches (Hook et al., 2014). However, in a 20-week randomized clinical trial of 54 gay or bisexual men, supportive group therapy demonstrated reductions in hypersexual symptoms (Quadland, 1985). In addition, individual acceptance and commitment psychotherapy demonstrated reductions in hypersexual symptoms during a manualized 12-week randomized clinical trial of 28 men presenting with hypersexual symptoms (Crosby, 2011).

In a single group study of hypersexual disorder, experiential psychotherapy showed reductions in hypersexual symptoms over time in a sample of 38 individuals (30 men and 8 women) (Klontz et al., 2005). A retrospective study of 138 individuals receiving cognitive behavior therapy in the form of an online psychoeducation program reported decreases in hypersexual sexual symptoms after a 26-week treatment period (Hardy et al., 2010). However, neither of these trials had a control arm.

Hypersexual behavior has shown an inverse relationship with mindfulness, suggesting that mindfulness training may be an effective psychotherapeutic aide in the treatment of patients with hypersexual disorder (Reid et al., 2014). The study examined the responses of a sample of 40 male patients with hypersexual disorder who had completed the HBI, the NEO Personality Inventory-Revised, and the Freiburg Mindfulness Inventory compared to the responses of 30 control participants (Reid et al., 2014).

Relapse prevention techniques have been suggested to treat paraphilic disorders and sexual addictions; psychodynamic psychotherapy has been suggested to assist patients in exploring family-of-origin, trauma, self-esteem, and identity issues; and couples therapy has been recommended to manage the interpersonal conflicts and effects of hypersexual disorder on the patient's partner and their relationship (Kaplan and Krueger, 2010). Twelve-step programs have been suggested as supplements to psychotherapy interventions in supporting patients through the recovery process and keeping them accountable for their behaviors (Kaplan and Krueger, 2010). However, more evidence is needed to demonstrate the efficacy of these interventions.

Research on the treatment of hypersexual disorder is at its initial stages, and although some pharmacotherapy and psychotherapy treatment trials have been conducted on small, predominantly male samples, more rigorous research is needed that draws from larger, more representative samples including women, sexual minorities, and different racial/ethnic groups. No medication is currently approved by regulatory agencies for the treatment of this condition.

FUTURE DIRECTIONS

There is growing recognition of hypersexual disorder in the literature. At the same time, differentiating hypersexual behavior from normal sexual behavior remains a challenge in the absence of a consensus about the optimal terminology and defining features of the disorder. Additional controversies arise in relation to our understanding of the pathogenesis and treatment of this condition. Establishment of a psychiatric diagnosis of "hypersexual disorder" or "compulsive sexual disorder" holds potential to provide a set of agreed upon clinical criteria, terminology, and features. Such a consensus may in turn encourage epidemiological and clinical research, ultimately improving the quality of research about hypersexual disorder as well as its treatment. The diagnosis would also arguably

encourage the development of standardized instruments to assess nosological criteria and symptom severity.

At this stage, there is insufficient empirical evidence to support any
particular pathophysiological model of hypersexual disorder or specific
criteria for assessment. Although further empirical research is needed,
each of these theoretical models has contributed to a fuller understanding of hypersexual disorder. Nevertheless, each model is associated with
different terminology and assessment tools, making it difficult to reach
consensus in the field. This lack of consensus may result in differing diagnoses and treatment plans. Although some empirical research is available,
more is needed, particularly with respect to understanding the clinical
course of the disorder, developmental risk factors, family history, neurobiology, and treatment. Methodologically rigorous controlled treatment
trials, and studies that include sufficient representation of women, sexual
minorities, and different racial or ethnic groups, are also lacking.

Although much remains to be learned about hypersexual behavior, its
diagnosis, and its treatment, a clinical population clearly exists for which
high frequency and intensity of sexual behaviors leads to significant distress and impairment in life functioning. The consequences of hypersexual
disorder include increased risk-taking behavior and STIs, interpersonal
difficulties, excessive financial expenses, and work or education concerns.
Whether the constellation of symptoms is best conceptualized as a sexual
desire dysregulation model, behavioral addition, an impulsive disorder,
or a combined ABC model remains an area of debate. Consensus on
the defining clinical criteria, terminology, and features would arguably
encourage the epidemiological and clinical research needed to improve
prevention and treatment options for these individuals.

REFERENCES

American Psychiatric Association, 1980. Diagnostic and statistical manual of mental
disorders (3rd ed.). Washington, DC: American Psychiatric Association.
American Psychiatric Association, 1986. Diagnostic and statistical manual of mental
disorders (3rd ed. rev.). Washington, DC: American Psychiatric Association.

American Psychiatric Association, 2013. Diagnostic and statistical manual of mental disorders (5th ed.). Washington, DC: American Psychiatric Association.

Bancroft, J., Graham, C.A., Janssen, E., Sanders, S., 2009. The dual control model: Current status and future directions. J Sex Res. 46, 121–142.

Black, D.W., Kehrberg, L.L., Flumerfelt, D.L., Schlosser, S.S., 1997. Characteristics of 36 subjects reporting compulsive sexual behavior. Am J Psychiatry. 154(2), 243–249.

Carnes, P., 1983. Out of the shadows: Understanding sexual addiction. Minneapolis, MN: CompCare.

Carnes, P., 1989. Contrary to love. Minneapolis, MN: Hazelden Foundation.

Carnes P., 1991. Don't call it love: Recovery from sexual addiction. New York: Bantam.

Carnes, P.J., Delmonico, D.L., 1996. Childhood abuse and multiple addictions: Research findings in a sample of self-identified sexual addicts. Sex Addict Compulsivity. 3, 258–268.

Coleman, E., Miner, M., Ohlerking, F., Raymond, N., 2001. Compulsive Sexual Behavior Inventory: A preliminary study of reliability and validity. J Sex Marital Ther. 27, 325–332.

Crosby, J.M., 2011. Acceptance and commitment therapy for the treatment of compulsive pornography use: A randomized clinical trial. Unpublished doctoral dissertation, Utah State University, Logan, UT.

Giugliano, J.R., 2013. Sex addiction as a mental health diagnosis: Coming together or coming apart. Sexologies. 22, 77–80.

Goodman, A., 2008. Neurobiology of addiction: An integrative review. Biochem Pharmacol. 75, 266–322.

Grant, J.E., Kim, S.W., 2003. Comorbidity of impulse control disorders in pathological gamblers. Acta Psychiatr Scand. 108(3), 203–207.

Grant, J.E., Steinberg, M.A., 2005. Compulsive sexual behavior and pathological gambling. Sex Addict Compulsivity. 12, 235–244.

Grant, J.E., Atmaca, M., Fineberg, N.A., Fontenelle, L.F., Matsunaga, H., Reddy, Y.C.J., et al., 2014. Internet and other proposed addictive behaviors in the International Classification of Diseases-11. World Psychiatry. 13(2), 125–127.

Hardy, S.A., Ruchty, J., Hull, T.D., Hyde, R., 2010. A preliminary study of an online psychoeducational program for hypersexuality. Sex Addict Compulsivity. 17, 247–269.

Hartmann, U.H., 2013. Re: Report of findings in a DSM-5 field trial for hypersexual disorder. Eur Urol. 64(4), 685–686.

Hook, J.N., Reid, R.C., Penberthy, J.K., Davis, D.E., & Jennings, D.J., 2014. Methodological review of treatments for nonparaphilic hypersexual behavior. Journal of Sex & Marital Therapy. 40(4), 294–308.

Janssen, E., Vorst, H., Finn, P., Bancroft, J., 2002a. The Sexual Inhibition (SIS) and Sexual Excitation (SES) Scales: I. Measuring sexual inhibition and excitation proneness in men. J Sex Res. 39, 114–126.

Janssen, E., Vorst, H., Finn, P., Bancroft, J., 2002b. The Sexual Inhibition (SIS) and Sexual Excitation (SES) Scales: II. Predicting psychophysiological response patterns. J Sex Res. 39, 127–132.

Kafka, M.P., 1997. Hypersexual desire in males: An operational definition and clinical implications for men with paraphilias and paraphilia-related disorders. Arch Sex Behav. 26, 505–526.

Kafka, M.P., 2010. Hypersexual disorder: A proposed diagnosis for DSM-V. Arch Sex Behav. 39(2), 377–400.

Kafka, M.P., Prentky, R., 1992. A comparative study of nonparaphilic sexual addictions and paraphilias in men. J Clin Psychiatry. 53(10) 345–350.

Kalichman, S.C., Rompa, D., 1995. Sexual Sensation Seeking and Sexual Compulsivity Scales: Reliability, validity, and predicting HIV risk behavior. J Pers Assess. 65, 586–601.

Kalichman, S.C., Johnson, J.R., Adair, V., Rompa, D., Multhauf, K., Kelley, J.A., 1994. Sexual sensation seeking: Scale development and predicting AIDS-risk behavior among homosexually active men. J Pers Assess. 62, 385–397.

Kaplan, M.S., Krueger, R.B., 2010. Diagnosis, assessment, and treatment of hypersexuality. J Sex Res. 47(2–3), 181–198.

Kingston, D.A., Firestone, P., 2008. Problematic hypersexuality: A review of conceptualization and diagnosis. Sex Addict Compulsivity. 15, 284–310.

Kinsey, A.C., Pomeroy, W.B., Martin, C.E., 1948. Sexual behavior in the human male. Philadelphia: Saunders.

Klontz, B.T., Garos, S., Klontz, P.T., 2005. The effectiveness of brief multimodal experiential therapy in the treatment of sexual addiction. Sex Addict Compulsivity. 12, 275–294.

Kor, A., Fogel, Y., Reid, R.C., Potensa, M.N., 2013. Should hypersexual disorder be classified as an addiction? Sex Addict Compulsivity. 20(1–2), 27–47.

Kruesi, M.J.P., Fine, S., Valladares, L., Phillips, R.A., Rapoport, J.L., 1992. Paraphilias: A double-blind crossover comparison of clomipramine versus desipramine. Arch Sex Behav. 21, 587–593.

Kuzma, J.M., Black, D.W., 2008. Epidemiology, prevalence, and natural history of compulsive sexual behavior. Psychiatr Clin North Am. 31(4), 603–611.

Långström, N., Hanson, R.K., 2006. High rates of sexual behavior in the general population: Correlates and predictors. Arch Sex Behav. 35, 37–52.

Laumann, E.O., Gagnon, J.H., Michael, R.T., Michaels, S., 1994. The social organization of sexuality: Sexual practices in the United States. Chicago: University of Chicago Press.

Lochner, C., Stein, D.J., 2010. Obsessive–compulsive spectrum disorders in obsessive–compulsive disorder and other anxiety disorders. Psychopathology. 43(6), 389–396.

Marshall, L.E., Briken, P., 2010. Assessment, diagnosis and management of hypersexual disorder. Curr Opin Psychiatry. 23(6), 570–573.

Marshall, L.E., Marshall, W.L., 2006. Sexual addiction in incarcerated sexual offenders. Sex Addict Compulsivity. 13(4), 377–390.

Quadland, M.C., 1985. Compulsive sexual behavior: Definition of a problem and an approach to treatment. J Sex Marital Ther. 11, 121–132.

Raymond, N.C., Coleman, E., Miner, M.H., 2003. Psychiatric comorbidity and compulsive/impulsive traits in compulsive sexual behavior. Compr Psychiatry. 44(5), 370–80.

Reid, R.C., Garos, S., Carpenter, B.N., 2011. Reliability, validity, and psychometric development of the Hypersexual Behavioral Inventory in an outpatient sample of men. Sex Addict Compulsivity. 18, 30–51.

Reid, R.C., Carpenter, B.N., Hook, J.N., Garos, S., Manning, J.C., Gilliland, R., et al., 2012. Report of findings in a DSM-V field trial for hypersexual disorder. J Sex Med. 9, 2826–2877.

Reid, R. C., Carpenter, B. N., Lloyd, T. Q., 2009. Assessing psychological symptom patterns of patients seeking help for hypersexual behavior. Sexual and Relationship Therapy. 24(1), 47–63.

Reid, R.C., Bramen, J.E., Anderson, A., Cohen, M.S., 2014. Mindfulness, emotional dysregulation, impulsivity and stress proneness among hypersexual patients. J Clin Psychol. 70, 313–321.

Rosenberg, K.P., Curtis Feder, L., 2014. An introduction to behavior addiction. In: Rosenberg, K.P., Curtis Feder, L. (Eds.), Behavioral addictions: Criteria, evidence and treatment (pp. 1–17). London: Academic Press.

Rosenberg, K.P., Carnes, P., O'Connor, S., 2013. Evaluation and treatment of sex addiction. J Sex Marital Ther. 40(2), 77–91.

Rosenberg, K.P., O'Connor, S., Carnes, P., 2014. Sex addiction: An overview. In: Rosenberg, K.P., Curtis Feder, L. (Eds.), Behavioral addictions: Criteria, evidence and treatment (pp. 215–233). London: Academic Press.

Schneider, J.P., Schneider, B.H., 1996. Couple recovery from sexual addiction: Research findings of a survey of 88 marriages. Sex Addict Compulsivity. 3, 111–126.

Schultz, K., Hook, J.N., Davis, D.E., Penberthy, J.K., Reid, R.C., 2014. Nonparaphilic hypersexual behavior and depressive symptoms: A meta-analytic review of the literature. J Sex Marital Ther. 40, 477–487.

Stein, D.J., 2008. Classifying hypersexual disorders: Compulsive, impulsive, and addictive models. Psychiatr Clin North Am. 31(4), 587–591.

Stein, D.J., Hollander, E., Anthony, D.T., Schneier, F.R., Fallon, B.A., Liebowitz, M.R., et al., 1992. Seotonergic medications for sexual obsessions, sexual addictions, and paraphilias. J Clin Psychiatry. 53(8), 267–271.

Stein, D.J., Hugo, F., Oosthuizen, P., Hawkridge, S.M., van Heerden, B., 2000. Neuropsychiatry of hypersexuality. CNS Spectr. 5(1), 36–46.

Wainberg, M.L., Muench, F., Morgenstern, J., Hollander, E., Irwin, T.W., Parsons, J.T., et al., 2006. A double-blind study of citalopram versus placebo in the treatment of compulsive sexual behaviors in gay and bisexual men. J Clin Psychiatry. 67, 1968–1973.

World Health Organization, 2007. International classification of diseases (10th ed.). Geneva: World Health Organization.

Zietsch, B.P., Verweij, K.J.H., Bailey, J.M., Wright, M.J., Martin, N.G., 2010. Genetics and environmental influences on risky sexual behaviour and its relationship with personality. Behav Genet. 40, 12–21.

6

Compulsive Shopping as a Behavioral Addiction

DONALD W. BLACK ■

Compulsive shopping (CS) behavior has been described for centuries among the wealthy and powerful. Some of the famous names throughout history associated with excessive buying behavior include Marie Antoinette, Mary Todd Lincoln, William Randolph Hearst, and Jaqueline Kennedy Onassis (Baker, 1987; Castelot, 1957; Erickson, 1991; Heymann, 1989; Swanberg, 1961). Whether these individuals were compulsive shoppers is unknown, yet each was reported to have episodes of senseless spending that contributed to their financial or personal difficulties. However, most compulsive shoppers are not famous or wealthy but, rather, are ordinary people whose excessive shopping has become an irresistible and costly way of life.

The first clinical description of CS was given by German psychiatrist Emil Kraepelin (1915), who wrote about the uncontrolled shopping and spending behavior of "buying maniacs." He was later quoted by the Swiss psychiatrist Eugen Bleuler (1930):

As a last category, Kraepelin mentions the buying maniacs (oniomaniacs) in whom even buying is compulsive and leads to senseless contraction of debts with continuous delay of payment until a catastrophe clears the situation a little—a little bit never altogether because they never admit all their debts. According to Kraepelin, here, too, it always involves women. ... The particular element is impulsiveness; they cannot help it, which sometimes even expresses itself in the fact that notwithstanding a good school intelligence, the patients are absolutely incapable to think differently and to conceive the senseless consequences of their act, and the possibilities of not doing it. (p. 540)

Kraepelin and Bleuler each considered "buying mania" a *reactive impulse* or *impulsive insanity* and grouped it with kleptomania and pyromania.

Despite this early work, CS attracted little attention except for occasional reports in the psychoanalytic literature (Krueger, 1988; Lawrence, 1990; Stekel, 1924; Winestine, 1985). Interest was rekindled in the late 1980s and early 1990s by consumer behavior researchers who showed the disorder to be widespread (Elliott, 1994; Magee, 1994; O'Guinn & Faber, 1989), and descriptive studies began to appear in the psychiatric literature (Christenson et al., 1994; McElroy et al., 1991, 1994; Schlosser et al., 1994). These reports were consistent in presenting a picture of an identifiable clinical disorder that mainly affected women, impaired psychosocial functioning, and caused considerable distress.

DEFINING FEATURES AND METHODS FOR ASSESSMENT

McElroy et al. (1994) developed operational criteria for CS that emphasize cognitive and behavioral aspects of the disorder. Their definition requires evidence of impairment from marked subjective distress, interference in social or occupational functioning, or financial/legal problems. Furthermore, the disorder cannot be attributed to mania or hypomania. These criteria have been embraced by researchers, but neither their reliability nor their validity has been established. Some writers have criticized attempts to categorize CS as an illness, which they view as part of a trend to "medicalize" behavioral problems (Lee and Mysyk, 2004). CS is not included in contemporary diagnostic systems, such as the the fifth edition of the *Diagnostic and Statistical Manual of Mental Disorders* (DSM-5; American Psychiatric Association, 2013) or the *International Classification of Diseases* (10th ed.; World Health Organization, 2007).

Other definitions have come from consumer behavior researchers or social psychologists. Faber and O'Guinn (1992) defined the disorder as "chronic buying episodes of a somewhat stereotyped fashion in which the consumer feels unable to stop or significantly moderate his behavior" (p. 738). Edwards (1993), another consumer behaviorist, suggested that compulsive buying is an "abnormal form of shopping and spending in which the afflicted consumer has an overpowering uncontrollable, chronic and repetitive urge to shop and spend [that functions] ... as a means of alleviating negative feelings of stress and anxiety" (p. 67). Dittmar (2004) considered irresistible impulse, loss of control, and carrying on despite adverse consequences as cardinal features of the disorder.

The appropriate classification of CS remains elusive. McElroy et al. (1991) suggested that compulsive shopping behavior might be related to "mood, obsessive–compulsive or impulse control disorders." Hollander (1993) later described a spectrum of disorders that he has connected to obsessive–compulsive disorders including CS, whereas Lejoyeux et al. (1996) linked it with mood disorders. Others consider CS to be related to the addictive disorders such as alcohol and drug dependence (Glatt and Cook, 1987; Goldman, 2000; Hartson, 2012; Krych, 1989).

More recently, CS has been conceptualized as a *behavioral addiction* (Hollander and Allen, 2006; Muller et al., 2013). Depending on the writer, this category potentially includes gambling disorder, kleptomania, pyromania, CS, Internet addiction, and compulsive sexual behavior. The National Institute on Drug Abuse considers behavioral addictions to be relatively pure models of addiction because they are not contaminated by the presence of an exogenous substance (Holden, 2001). Di Nicola et al. (2010) have described an association between bipolar disorder and behavioral addictions. In several respects, CS is not dissimilar from substance addictions because both involve excessive or poorly controlled behaviors, cravings, and preoccupation (Goldman, 2000). Of course, the unique behavioral aspect of CS is the object of the craving or preoccupations: shopping.

The hallmark of CS is the individual's preoccupation with shopping and spending. Many hours may be devoted each week to these behaviors (Christenson et al., 1994; Schlosser et al., 1994). Persons with CS often describe anxiety and tension relieved by making a purchase. CS behaviors occur year-round but can be more problematic during Christmas, other holidays, and special days such as birthdays of family members and friends.

People with CS show a range of behavior regarding the outcome of a purchase: returning the item, failing to remove the item from the package, selling the item, or even giving it away (Schlosser et al., 1994). CS tends to be a private experience, so individuals with CS prefer to shop alone (Schlosser et al., 1994). Compulsive shopping can occur in any venue: high-fashion department stores and boutiques, consignment shops, garage sales, or catalogs (Christenson et al., 1994). Dittmar (2007) documented how CS has gained a strong foothold with online buying. People with CS are mainly interested in consumer goods such as clothing, shoes, crafts, jewelry, gifts, makeup, and audio recordings (e.g., CDs/DVDs) (Christenson et al., 1994; Mitchell et al., 2006; Schlosser et al., 1994).

Some individuals with CS have an intense interest in new clothing styles and products. They may report buying a product based on its attractiveness or because it was a "bargain" (Frost et al., 1998). Individually, items purchased tend not to be large or expensive, but many compulsive shoppers will buy in quantity so that spending rapidly escalates. During a typical episode, compulsive shoppers have reported spending an average of $110 (Christenson et al., 1994), $92 (Schlosser et al., 1994), or $89 (Miltenberger et al., 2003). Compulsive buying disorder has little to do with intellect or educational level and has been observed to occur in mentally retarded persons (Otter & Black, 2007).

Several writers have emphasized the emotional significance of the types of objects purchased, which may address personal and social identity needs (Dittmar, 2007; Richards, 1996). Richards stressed the role of clothing in developing a feminine identity and noted that voids in one's identity have their roots in failed parent–child interactions. Krueger (1988) observed that emotionally deprived persons unconsciously replace what is missing with objects in an attempt to "fill the emptiness of depression and the absence of self-regulation" (p. 582). These explanations for compulsive buying behaviors may apply to some but certainly not all persons with CS. One relevant study found that self-image concerns were more closely linked to the motivations underlying CS in women than in men (Dittmar and Drury, 2000).

Miltenberger et al. (2003) reported that negative emotions, such as anger, anxiety, boredom, and self-critical thoughts, were the most common antecedents to shopping binges in a group of persons with CS; euphoria or relief of negative emotions has been the most common immediate emotional reaction (Elliott et al., 1996). Lejoyeux et al. (1996) concluded that for some persons, "uncontrolled buying, like bulimia, can be used as a compensatory mechanism for depressive feelings" (p. 1528). Faber and Christenson (1996) commented on the close relationships among shopping, self-esteem, and negative emotions. Faber (1992) concluded that shopping behavior is likely to become problematic when it provides a sense of recognition and acceptance for people with low self-esteem, allowing them to act out anger or aggression while providing an escape from their day-to-day drudgery.

Nataraajan and Goff (1991) identified two independent factors in CS: (1) buying urge or desire and (2) degree of control over buying. In their model, compulsive shoppers combine high urge with low control. This view is consistent with clinical reports that compulsive buyers are preoccupied with shopping and spending and will try to resist their urges but often have little success (Black, 2001; Christenson et al., 1994). For example, in the study of Christenson et al., 92% of persons with CS described attempts to resist urges to buy but reported that their attempts were often unsuccessful. Subjects indicated that the urge to buy resulted in a purchase 74% of the time. Typically, 1 to 5 hours passed between initially experiencing the urge to buy and the eventual purchase.

Clinical reports suggest that the disorder is chronic or episodic. Schlosser et al. (1994) reported that 59% of their subjects described their course as continuous and 41% as episodic. Of the 20 subjects described in the study of McElroy et al. (1994), 60% had a chronic course, whereas 8% described an episodic course. In a medication study, Aboujaoude et al. (2003) suggested that persons who responded to treatment with citalopram were likely to remain in remission during a 1-year follow-up period. Mueller et al. (2008) similarly reported that treatment with group cognitive–behavior therapy led to improvement that was maintained during a 6-month follow-up period. These studies suggest that treatment may alter the natural history of the disorder.

The initial goal of evaluation is to determine if the patient has a shopping disorder. If confirmed, the clinician can inquire about the person's attitudes about shopping and spending, and he or she can then focus on specific shopping behaviors and patterns. For most persons with CS, preoccupation with shopping and spending is a hallmark of the disorder (Black, 2001). For general screening purposes, a clinician might ask the following:

- Do you feel overly preoccupied with shopping and spending?
- Do you ever feel that your shopping behavior is excessive, inappropriate, or uncontrolled?
- Have your shopping desires, urges, fantasies, or behaviors ever been overly time-consuming, caused you to feel upset or guilty, or led to serious problems in your life (e.g., financial or legal problems, relationship loss)?

A positive response should be followed up with more detailed questions about shopping and spending. Family members and friends can become important informants in the assessment of CS by filling in gaps in the patient's history or describing the patient's behavior they may have witnessed.

In considering a diagnosis of CS, the patient's pattern of shopping and spending must be distinguished from normal buying behavior. Because shopping is a major pastime for people in the United States and other developed countries (Farrell, 2003), frequent shopping does not by itself constitute evidence in support of a CS. For the person with CS, the frequent shopping and spending have a compulsive and irresistible quality and lead to deleterious consequences. Normal buying can take on a compulsive quality, particularly around the time of special holidays or birthdays, but the excessive buying is not persistent, nor does it lead to distress or impairment. People who receive an inheritance or win a lottery may experience shopping sprees as well. The clinician should exercise judgment in applying the diagnostic criteria of McElroy et al. (1994) and be mindful of the need for evidence of distress or impairment.

Several instruments have been developed to help identify and diagnose CS. Canadian researchers Valence et al. (1988) developed the Compulsive Buying Measurement Scale. Starting with 16 items thought to represent four basic dimensions of compulsive buying (a tendency to spend, feeling an urge to buy or shop, post-purchase guilt, and family environment), the list was pared to 13 items based on a reliability analysis; the remaining items had high internal consistency. Construct validity was established by demonstrating that those with CS achieved significantly higher scores than the control group, and the higher scores correlated with higher levels of anxiety and with having a family history of psychiatric illness. A modified version of the scale containing 16 items, each rated on a 4-point scale, was tested by German researchers (Scherhorn et al., 1990). Their Addictive Buying Indicator was found to have high reliability (Cronbach's alpha = .87); construct validity was demonstrated by significant correlations between scale scores and scores assessing psychasthenia, depression, and self-esteem. Like the Canadian instrument, the Addictive Buying Indicator was able to discriminate individuals with normal shopping behaviors from individuals with CS.

These efforts led Faber and O'Guinn (1992) to develop the Compulsive Buying Scale (CBS), an instrument designed to identify people with CS. They began with 29 items based on preliminary work, and each was rated on a 5-point scale chosen to reflect important characteristics of compulsive buying. Their scale was administered to 388 self-identified compulsive buyers and 292 persons drawn randomly from the general population. Using logistic regression, 7 items representing specific behaviors, motivations, and feelings associated with buying significantly were found to correctly classify approximately 88% of the subjects. The CBS also showed excellent reliability and validity. One measure of reliability, internal consistency, was verified using principal components factor analysis as well as by calculating Cronbach's alpha (.95). Criterion and construct validity were assessed by comparing compulsive buyers from the general population sample (classified by the screener) to the self-identified compulsive buyers and to the other members of the general population on variables previously found to relate to compulsive buying (Faber and O'Guinn, 1989). The comparison provides good support for the validity of the screener. This instrument has become a gold standard in CS research.

Christenson et al. (1994) developed the Minnesota Impulsive Disorder Interview (MIDI) to assess the presence of CS, kleptomania, trichotillomania, intermittent explosive disorder, pathological gambling, compulsive sexual behavior, and compulsive exercise. This diagnostic instrument is fully structured and designed for use in research settings. The MIDI begins by gathering demographic data and then progresses through various screening modules. It is followed by a section on family history and personality characteristics. The section on compulsive buying consists of four core questions and five follow-up questions. The developers recommend administering their 82-question expanded module to persons screening positive for compulsive buying. Expanded modules are also available for trichotillomania and compulsive sexual behavior. Grant et al. (2005) reported that the instrument had a sensitivity of 100% and a specificity of 96.2% for CS when comparing the instrument to the diagnostic criteria of McElroy et al. (1994).

Edwards (1993) and DeSarbo and Edwards (1996) have developed a 13-item self-report scale designed to identify persons with CS behavior and to rate its severity. Each item is rated on a 5-point Likert-like scale. In a study comparing the responses of 104 people with CS recruited through support groups and 101 persons from the general population, the authors identified five factors constituting compulsive spending: compulsion/drive to spend, feelings about shopping and spending, tendency to spend, dysfunctional spending, and post-purchase guilt. Based on their results, the authors pared the scale to 13 items. The scale and its subscales showed good to excellent internal consistency as estimated by Cronbach's alpha (range, .76–.91).

Lejoyeux et al. (1997) developed a questionnaire consisting of 19items that tap the basic features of CS. These dimensions include impulsivity; urges to shop and buy; emotions felt before, during, and after purchasing; post-purchase guilt and regret; degree of engagement of short-term gratification; tangible consequences of buying; and avoidance strategies. Its psychometric properties have not been examined.

Weun et al. (1998) developed the Impulse Buying Tendency Scale to assess the proclivity for impulse buying, which they distinguish from compulsive buying. Ridgeway et al. (2008) developed the Compulsive–Impulsive Buying Scale, which measures compulsive buying as a construct incorporating elements of both an obsessive–compulsive and an impulse–control disorder. The scale appears to be reliable and valid, and it performs well in correlating with other theoretically related constructs.

Monahan et al. (1996) modified the Yale–Brown Obsessive–Compulsive Scale (YBOCS) (Goodman et al., 1989) to create the YBOCS-Shopping Version (YBOCS-SV) to assess cognitions and behaviors associated with compulsive buying. The authors concluded that their scale is reliable and valid in measuring severity and change during clinical trials. The developers compared a group of clinically identified compulsive buyers and control subjects and showed that the scale separated the two groups and exhibited high inter-rater reliability. The instrument also showed a high degree of internal consistency, and evidence for construct validity was good as well; YBOCS-SV scores were the best indicators of severity of illness of CS, not other scales that were administered, including the Clinical Global Impression Scales (Guy, 1976) and the National Institutes of Mental Health Obsessive–Compulsive Scale (Murphy et al., 1982). The YBOCS-SV was sensitive to clinical change and was able to detect improvement during a clinical trial (Black et al., 1997, 2000).

The YBOCS-SV consists of 10 items, 5 of which rate preoccupations and 5 that rate behaviors. For assessing both preoccupations and behaviors, subjects are asked about time involved, interference due to the preoccupations or behaviors, distress associated with shopping, the resistance to the thoughts or behavior, and degree of control over the symptoms. Items are rated from 0 (none) to 4 (extreme), and scores can range from 0 to 40. In the sample described by Monahan et al. (1996), the mean YBOCS-SV score for untreated compulsive shoppers was 21 (range, 18–25), and it was 4 (range, 1–7) for normal shoppers. This instrument has become standard for use in clinical trials.

Any effort to understand and treat CS will benefit by having individuals keep a daily log of their shopping and spending behavior: where they shop, how much they spend, and what they buy. It also may be helpful to have patients record their mood at the time and to note whether the buying episode was prompted by anything in particular. The data collected can be used to gain a sense of the person's typical buying behavior, as well as to provide data that can be directly monitored during a treatment trial. The data can be used to supplement (and externally validate) the rating scale scores. Benson (2008) described how shopping diaries can be embedded within a self-help program.

PREVALENCE RATES

Prevalence surveys provide rates for CS that range from 1.4% to 44%. The wide range is likely due to differences in the populations examined and the research methods used (Table 6.1). In one of the first studies, Faber and O'Guinn (1992) estimated the prevalence of CS at between 1.8% and 8.1% of the general population based on results from a mail survey. The CBS (Faber and O'Guinn, 1989) was given to 292 individuals who were selected to approximate the demographic makeup of the general population of Illinois. The high and low prevalence estimates reflect different thresholds (or cut-points) set for compulsive buying disorder (CBD). The higher percentage is based on a probability level of .70 (i.e., two standard deviations above the mean). The lower percentage is based on a more conservative probability level of .95 (i.e., three standard deviations above the mean). These authors recommend using the probability level of .70 with the CBS.

Dittmar (2005) queried 194 persons who responded to an unsolicited mail survey and were residentially matched to a group of persons with

Table 6.1 PREVALENCE SURVEYS OF COMPULSIVE SHOPPING

Study	Location	Diagnostic Method	Sample Size	Setting	Findings
Faber and O'Guinn (1992)[a]	Illinois	CBS	292	General population	1.8%/ 8.1%
Magee (1994)	Arizona	CBS	94	College students	16%
Hassay and Smith (1996)	Manitoba, Canada	CBS	92	College students	12%
Roberts (1998)	Texas	CBS	300	College students	6%
Dittmar (2005)	England	CBS	194	General population	13.5%
Dittmar (2005)	England	CBS	195	Adolescents	44.1%
Neuner et al. (2005)[b]	Germany	ABS	1,527/ 1,017	General population	6.5%/ 8%
Grant et al. (2005)	Minnesota	MIDI	204	Psychiatric inpatient unit	9.5%
Koran et al. (2006)[a]	United States	CBS	2,513	General population	1.4%/ 5.8%

[a]The study used conservative and liberal cut-points with the CBS.
[b]The study involved interviews with East and West Germans in 1991/2001.
ABS, Addictive Buying Scale; CBS, Compulsive Buying Scale; MIDI, Minnesota Impulsive Disorders Interview.

shopping problems. Using the CBS, she found that 13.4% of persons in the comparison group met the threshold for CS. She also sampled 195 adolescents aged 16 to 18 years and found that 44.1% scored above the CBS scale threshold, indicating the presence of CS. Koran et al. (2006) used the CBS to identify people with CS in a random telephone survey of 2,513 U.S. adults and estimated the point prevalence at 5.8% of respondents. The estimate was calculated by using CBS scores two standard deviations above the mean. A prevalence of 1.4% was calculated using the stricter criterion of three standard deviations above the mean.

In general, adolescents and young adults have higher rates of CS than those of adult populations. Magee (1994) reported that 16% of 94 undergraduates had CS, compared to 12.2% reported by Hassay and Smith (1996) in 92 undergraduates and 6% of 300 college students (Roberts, 1998). A study of high school students in southern Italy found that 11% had CS behavior (Villella et al., 2011), whereas an online survey of college students in the United States was assessed using the Minnesota Impulsive Disorders Interview (described later) and found a rate for CS of 3.5% of 2,108 respondents (Harvanko et al., 2013).

In the clinical setting, Grant et al. (2005) utilized the Minnesota Impulsive Disorders Interview (Christenson et al., 1994) to assess CS and reported a lifetime prevalence of 9.3% among 204 consecutively admitted psychiatric inpatients.

In an interesting study, Neuner et al. (2005) addressed the question of whether CS prevalence is increasing. They reported that from 1991 to 2001, the frequency of CS in Germany increased. Using the Addictive Buying Scale, these investigators found that the frequency of CS increased from 1% to 6.5% in eastern Germany and from 5% to 8% in western Germany. They attributed the rapid rise of CS in the former East Germany in part to the acculturation process brought about by reunification.

COMORBIDITIES WITH OTHER PSYCHIATRIC DISORDERS

Data from clinical studies confirm high rates of major mental disorders in persons with CS (Table 6.2), particularly mood (21%–100%), anxiety (41%–87%), substance use (21%–46%), impulse control disorders (21%–69%), and eating disorders (0%–35%). Four clinical studies included comparison groups: (1) Black et al. (1998) reported that major depression and "any" mood disorder were excessive; (2) Christenson et al. (1994) reported that the categories of anxiety, substance use, eating, and impulse control disorders were each excessive; (3) Mueller et al. (2009) found that persons with CS had higher rates of mood, anxiety, and eating disorders than community controls and also higher rates of mood and anxiety disorders

Table 6.2 Lifetime Psychiatric Comorbidity in Persons With Compulsive Shopping

Comorbid Disorder	Study First Author (Year)									
	Schlosser (1994)	Christenson (1994)	McElroy (1994)	Lejoyeux (1997)	Black (1998)	Ninan (2000)	Koran (2002)	Mitchell (2006)	Muller (2009)	Black (2012)
Instrument used	DIS	SCID	SCID	MINI	SCID	SCID	MINI	SCID	SCID	MINI
Mood disorder (%)	28	54	95	100	61	45	8	62	80	62
Anxiety disorder (%)	41	50	80	a	42			26	87	50
Substance use disorder (%)	30	46	40		21			33	23	23
Somatoform disorder (%)	11		10							12
Eating disorder (%)	17	21	35	21	15		8	18	33	0
Impulse control disorder (%)		21	40						20	69

DIS, Diagnostic Interview Schedule; MINI, Mini International Neuropsychiatric Interview; SCID, Structured Clinical Interview for DSM-IV.
[a]Blank cells indicate that the disorder was not assessed.

compared to bariatric controls; and (4) Black et al. (2012) reported that people with CS had higher rates of mood, anxiety, and impulse control disorders than matched community controls.

CS may have a special relationship with obsessive–compulsive disorder (OCD). In clinical samples, from 3% (Black et al., 1998) to 40% (Mueller et al., 2009) of individuals with CS are reported to have comorbid OCD. Likewise, the presence of CS may characterize a specific subset of OCD patients (du Toit et al., 2001; Hantouche et al., 1996, 1997), particularly those who hoard, a special symptom that involves the acquisition of, and failure to discard, possessions of limited use or value (Frost et al., 2001). Unlike the items kept by the typical hoarder, items purchased by the individual with CS are not inherently useless or lacking in value.

In perhaps the largest study to assess comorbidity, Mueller et al. (2010) pooled the data from 175 people with CS in the United States and Germany. (Because the pooled data were previously published, these results are not included in Table 6.2.) Nearly 90% of the subjects had at least one lifetime diagnosis, including mood (74%) and anxiety (57%) disorders. Half of the subjects had at least one current disorder, most commonly an anxiety disorder (40%). Twenty-one percent had a comorbid lifetime impulse control disorder, most commonly intermittent explosive disorder (11%).

Mueller et al. (2010) used latent profile analysis to identify clusters based on CS severity. The first cluster included nearly two-thirds of the total sample and was less symptomatic than the second cluster, which was characterized by more severe CS. Individuals in the second cluster had much higher rates of current and lifetime co-occurring psychiatric disorders than those in the first cluster. These data are partially compatible with the findings of Black et al. (2001), who divided a sample of 44 individuals with CS into four groups ranked from most to least severe based on their CBS score. Greater severity was associated with higher rates of psychiatric comorbidity. Those with more severe CS also had lower gross income, were less likely to have an income above the median, and spent a lower percentage of their income on sale items. Perhaps more severe buying disorders occur in individuals with low incomes with impaired ability to control or delay their urges to make inappropriate purchases and who have high rates of psychiatric comorbidity.

In one of the first studies of personality disorder prevalence in CS patients, Schlosser et al. (1994) found that nearly 60% of 46 persons recruited from the community met criteria for at least one personality disorder. The most commonly identified personality disorders were the obsessive–compulsive (22%), avoidant (15%), and borderline (15%) types. Mueller et al. (2008) examined 48 persons participating in a clinical trial and reported that depressive, avoidant, and obsessive–compulsive personality disorders were frequent. In a controlled study, Mueller et al. (2009) reported that 30 persons with CS had higher rates of personality disorders than community controls or bariatric clinic patients, particularly depressive, avoidant, obsessive–compulsive, and borderline types. Anecdotally, Krueger (1988) observed that the 4 patients he treated using psychoanalysis each exhibited aspects of narcissistic character pathology.

In terms of dimensional traits, Lejoyeux et al. (1997) reported that depressed people with CS had higher scores than depressed normal buyers on the experience-seeking subscale of the Zuckerman Sensation Seeking Scale (Zuckerman, 1994), as well as higher cognitive impulsivity, motor impulsivity, nonplanning activity, and total scores for the Barratt Impulsiveness Scale (Barratt, 1959). O'Guinn and Faber (1989) reported high levels of compulsivity, materialism, and fantasy but lower levels of self-esteem in compulsive buyers compared to normal buyers. Partially consistent with these results, Yurchistan and Johnson (2007) reported that compulsive buying behavior was negatively related to self-esteem and positively related to perceived social status associated with buying, materialism, and apparel-product acquisition. These findings suggest that many compulsive shoppers use possessions to boost their perceived social position, possibly in an attempt to boost low self-esteem. Otero-Lopez and Pol (2013) reported findings using the Five Factor model and CS from a population-based study. Those with a high propensity for CS had high levels of neuroticism but were low in conscientiousness and agreeableness.

Black et al. (2012) reported that compared to controls, a group of 32 people with CS had elevated levels of self-reported depression and symptoms of attention deficit hyperactivity disorder, trait impulsivity, and novelty seeking. However, comprehensive neuropsychological testing failed to differentiate those with CS from the controls, with the exception that individuals with CS performed better on the Wechsler Abbreviated Scale of Intelligence Picture Completion task, a test of visual perception. In contrast, Derbyshire et al. (2014) reported on 23 persons with CS who had problems in several distinct cognitive domains, including response inhibition, spatial working memory, and risk adjustment during decision-making. The authors suggest that these findings place CS alongside the alcohol and drug addictions.

RISK AND PROTECTIVE FACTORS

Community-based clinical studies, and the survey results of Faber and O'Guinn (1992), suggested that 80% to 94% of persons with CS are women. In contrast, Koran et al. (2006) reported that the prevalence of CS in their random telephone survey was nearly equal for men and women (5.5% and 6.0%, respectively). Their finding suggests that the reported gender difference may be spurious and is due to the fact that women more readily acknowledge abnormal shopping behavior than do men; women also are more willing to participate in research protocols. Based on the results of a general population survey in the United Kingdom, Dittmar (2004) concluded that the gender difference is real and not an artifact of men being underrepresented in clinical samples. The Internet-based survey by Harvanko et al. (2013) supports the conclusions of Dittmar. In this study of U.S. college students, these investigators found that significantly more women (4.4%) than men (2.5%) were affected.

Compulsive shopping has an onset in the late teens or early 20s, which may correspond with emancipation from the nuclear family (Table 6.3), as well as with the age at which people first establish credit (Black, 2001; Black et al., 2012). Roberts and Tanner (2000, 2002) showed that

Table 6.3 STUDIES INVOLVING PERSONS WITH COMPULSIVE SHOPPING

Investigators	Location	No. of Subjects	Age (Years, Mean)	% Female	Age at Onset (Years, Mean)	Duration of Illness (Years, Mean)
O'Guinn and Faber (1989)	Los Angeles, CA	386	37	92	N/A	N/A
Scherhorn et al. (1990)	Germany	26	40	85	N/A	N/A
McElroy et al. (1994)	Cincinnati, OH	20	39	80	30	9
Christenson et al. (1994)	Minneapolis, MN	24	36	92	18	18
Schlosser et al. (1994)	Iowa City, IA	46	31	80	19	12
Black et al. (1998)	Iowa City, IA	33	40	94	N/A	N/A
Ninan et al. (2000)	Cincinnati, OH; Boston, MA	42	41	81	N/A	N/A
Koran et al. (2002)	Stanford, CA	24	44	92	22	22
Miltenberger et al (2003)	Fargo, ND	19	N/A	100[a]	18	N/A
Mitchell et al. (2006)	Fargo, ND	39	45	100[a]	N/A	N/A
Mueller et al. (2008)	Bavaria, Germany	60	41	85	27	14
Black et al. (2012)	Iowa City, IA	32	36	88	20	17

[a]Indicates that the sample recruited was female.
N/A, not applicable.

uncontrolled buying in adolescents is associated with a more generalized pattern of behavioral disinhibition that includes smoking, alcohol and drug use, and early sex.

Research shows that CS adversely impacts the lives of those with the disorder and those of their family members. Most individuals with

CS admit that the disorder is subjectively distressing and that they feel unable to control their behavior (Christenson et al., 1994; Schlosser et al., 1994). They report that the disorder has led to marital and family problems, including separation and divorce. Financial problems that include substantial debt can lead to bankruptcy, and in some cases persons will turn to crime (e.g., embezzlement and shoplifting) to fuel their shopping or to repay their debts. Lejoyeux et al. (1997) reported that CS is associated with suicide attempts. There are no reports of CS leading to completed suicide.

In terms of family histories and genetics, McElroy et al. (1994) reported that of 18 individuals with CS, 17 had one or more first-degree relatives with major depression, 11 had an alcohol or other substance use disorder, 3 had an anxiety disorder, and 3 had relatives with CS. Black et al. (1998) used the family history method to assess 137 first-degree relatives of 31 persons with CS. Relatives were significantly more likely than those in a comparison group to have a depressive disorder, an alcohol disorder, or a drug use disorder. They were also more likely to have "any psychiatric disorder" and "more than one psychiatric disorder." CS was identified in 9.5% of the first-degree relatives but was not assessed in the comparison group. Recently, Black et al. (2015) reported results from a large family study which showed that first-degree relatives of people with pathological gambling have high rates of CS, a finding that suggests that the two disorders are related.

Two molecular genetic studies of CS have been published. Comings et al. (1997) found a significant correlation between polymorphism at the D1 receptor gene and the association of Tourette's disorder with gambling, alcohol abuse, and CS. Devor et al. (1999) were unable to find an association of CS to the serotonin transporter gene polymorphism.

Income has relatively little to do with CS. Level of income may lead one person to shop at a consignment shop, whereas another shops at a high-end boutique. Persons with a low income can be as preoccupied with shopping and spending as wealthier individuals (Black, 2001; Dittmar, 2007). Wealth also does not protect against CS because the presence of CS may cause or contribute to interpersonal, occupational, or marital problems even when it does not create financial or legal problems. Moreover, Koran et al. (2006) found that compared to other respondents, individuals with CS were more likely to report an income under $50,000, were less likely to pay off credit card balances in full, and gave maladaptive responses regarding their consumer behavior. In this study, compulsive buyers engaged in "problem shopping" more frequently and for longer periods and were more likely than other respondents to feel depressed after shopping, to make senseless and impulsive purchases, and to experience uncontrollable buying binges.

Because CS occurs mainly in developed countries, cultural and social factors have been proposed as either causing or promoting the disorder (Black, 2001; Dittmar, 2007). The disorder has been described worldwide, with reports from the United States (Christenson et al., 1994; McElroy et al., 1994; Schlosser et al., 1994), Australia (Kyrios et al., 2002), Brazil (Bernik et al., 1996), Canada (Valence et al., 1988), England (Dittmar, 2004; Elliott, 1994), Germany (Mueller et al., 2007; Scherhorn et al., 1990), France (Lejoyeux et al., 1997), The Netherlands (Otter and Black, 2007), Mexico (Roberts and Sepulveda, 1999), South Korea (Kwak et al., 2003), Spain (Villarino et al., 2001), and Taiwan (Lo and Harvey, 2011). In one cross-cultural study, Mueller et al. (2007) reported that a comparison of German and U.S. women with CS showed that the German women had higher rates of mood, anxiety, and somatoform disorders, but they did not differ with regard to severity of CS.

The presence of a market-based economy, the availability of a wide variety of goods, easily obtained credit, disposable income, and significant leisure time are elements that appear necessary for the development of CBD (Lee and Mysyk, 2004). A study in Europe and Taiwan showed the effect of credit card availability in fueling CS. The investigators (Lo and Harvey, 2011) found in an Internet-based study that overspending in respondents with CS was partially mediated by excessive use of credit cards.

Psychoanalysts have suggested that early life events, including childhood sexual abuse, contribute to the development of CS (Krueger, 1988; Lawrence, 1990; Stekel, 1924; Winestine, 1985). Benson (2008) observed several family constellations that she believes contribute to the development of CS: the physically abusive or neglectful parent, the emotionally neglectful parent who demands the child earn his or her love through "good" behavior, the absent parent who has little time or energy for the child, and families that have experienced financial reversals and fixate on lost luxury. In each scenario, possessions achieve importance as a means of easing suffering, boosting self-esteem, or restoring lost social status.

Neurobiologic theories have centered on disturbed neurotransmission, particularly involving the serotonergic, dopaminergic, or opioid systems. Selective serotonin reuptake inhibitors (SSRIs) have been used to treat CS (Black et al., 1997, 2000; Koran et al., 2003, 2007; Ninan et al., 2000), in part because of hypothetical similarities between CS and obsessive–compulsive disorder, a disorder known to respond to SSRIs (Hollander, 1993). Dopamine has been theorized to play a role in "reward dependence," which has been claimed to foster behavioral addictions such as CS and pathological gambling (Holden, 2001). Case reports suggesting benefit from the opiate antagonist naltrexone have led to speculation about the role of opiate receptors (Grant, 2003; Kim, 1998). There is no direct evidence, however, to support the role of these neurotransmitter systems in the etiology of CS.

In a study with relevance to CS, Knutson et al. (2007) used functional magnetic resonance imaging (fMRI) to explore neural circuits involved in purchasing decisions. The nucleus accumbens, a putative pleasure center, was activated when subjects were shown products they liked. When the item was priced lower than what the subject was willing to pay, the mesial prefrontal cortex (a brain region involved in decision-making) became activated, and the insula (a part of the brain that registers pain) showed less activity. The picture was reversed when the item was priced higher than what the subject was willing to pay. Subjects then made the decision to buy, with high mesial prefrontal cortex activity indicating a decision to buy and high insula activity indicating a decision to refrain. This study supports the view that consumers balance immediate pleasure (purchasing) against immediate pain (price). Although the subjects were drawn from the general population, the study may help to explain compulsive

shopping behavior: The pleasure of impulse buying is immediately registered, while the pain of delayed payment (i.e., from a credit card) is
minimized.

In the only relevant fMRI study, Raab et al. (2012) reported on differences between 23 persons with CS and 26 healthy consumers and
found greater nucleus accumbens activity during product presentation in
women with CS compared to those without and also lower insula activation during presentation of prices for the products the CS women decided
to purchase. The investigators concluded that the expected loss of money
did lead to a stronger negative emotional response in healthy controls
than in women with CS.

TREATMENTS

Several case studies report the psychoanalytic treatment of CS (Krueger,
1988; Lawrence, 1990; Schwartz, 1992; Stekel, 1924; Winestine, 1985).
Stekel described a woman whose CS was attributed to unconscious wishes
for sexual adventure. Three months of psychoanalysis left her sexually
responsive and free of her compulsive buying. Krueger described four
cases to show that the CS was motivated by a "dual attempt to regulate the
affect and fragmented sense of self and to restore self–object equilibrium,
symbolically or indirectly" (p. 583). None experienced clear-cut improvement from the therapy. Winestine presented the case of a woman with a
history of sexual abuse and fantasies of being the wife of a famous mil-
lionaire who had the power and funds to afford anything she wished. In
identifying with this role, she was thought to be reversing her actual feelings of helplessness and inability to regulate her shopping and spending
behavior: "The purchases offered some momentary fortification against
her feelings of humiliation and worthlessness for being out of control"
(p. 71). Lawrence wrote that compulsive shopping stems from an "intrapsychic need for nurturing from the external world" (p. 67); he may have
been the first mental health professional to link compulsive buying with
an attempt to deny death. Krueger (2000) described three additional

cases and wrote that compulsive shoppers have a fragile sense of self and self-esteem that depend on the responses of others. Goldman (2000) surmised that compulsive buying often follows the disruption of an emotional bond, setting into motion a desperate need to appear attractive and desirable. Benson and Gengler (2004), in considering the different forms of individual therapy, suggested that there are many different psychodynamic explanations of compulsive buying, usually related to the theoretical perspective of the therapist.

Cognitive–behavioral treatment (CBT) models have been developed for CS during approximately the past two decades. Lejoyeux et al. (1996) and Bernik et al. (1996) both suggested that cue exposure and response prevention may be helpful. Bernik et al. reported two patients with comorbid panic disorder and agoraphobia responsive to clomipramine, whose uncontrolled buying did not respond to the drug. Both patients responded well to 3 or 4 weeks of daily cue exposure and response prevention, although no follow-up data were presented.

The first use of group therapy for CS was described by Damon (1988). Later models were developed by Burgard and Mitchell (2000), Villarino et al. (2001), and Benson and Gengler (2004). Mitchell et al. (2006) found that group CBT (n = 28 subjects) produced significant improvement compared to a wait list (n = 11 subjects) in a 12-week pilot study. Improvement attributed to CBT was maintained during a 6-month follow-up. More recently, Benson et al. (2014) reported that a hybrid model that included elements of CBT, dialectical behavior therapy, psychodynamic psychotherapy, psychoeduction, and acceptance and commitment therapy was effective in 11 subjects compared to a wait list. The group therapy was based on a guided self-help program that that Benson (2006) had described earlier. The program includes a detailed workbook with text and exercises, a shopping diary for self-monitoring during shopping, a CD-ROM with guided visualizations, and a reminder card to be carried at all times.

McElroy et al. (1991) described 3 women with comorbid mood or anxiety disorders who had a partial or full remission of CS associated with fluoxetine, bupropion, or nortriptyline treatment. In a subsequent report, McElroy et al. (1994) described 20 additional patients, 9 of whom had partial or full remission during treatment with antidepressants, mainly serotonin reuptake inhibitors, usually in combination with a mood stabilizer. In most cases, the observation period was limited to a few weeks or months, and 2 of the patients who improved also received supportive or insight-oriented psychotherapy before receiving drug treatment. Lejoyeux et al. (1995) reported that treatment of depression in 2 patients with comorbid CS led to resolution of CS. In one case, clomipramine (150 mg/day) was used; in the other, no drug was specified.

Black et al. (1997) reported that 9 of 10 nondepressed subjects with CS given fluvoxamine in a 9-week, open-label trial showed benefit. Those who responded did so by Week 5. The fact that none were depressed appeared to refute the assertion by Lejoyeux et al. (1995) that the presence of comorbid depression explained the improvement in buying behavior during antidepressant treatment.

Two subsequent randomized controlled trials found fluvoxamine treatment no better than placebo. Black et al. (2000) randomized 12 nondepressed patients with CS to fluvoxamine and 11 to placebo. At the end of the 9-week trial, 50% of fluvoxamine recipients and 64% of placebo recipients had responded. There were no significant differences between the treatment groups on any of the main outcome measures in the intent-to-treat analysis. Similarly, in a 12-week, two-site trial in which 20 subjects received fluvoxamine and 17 placebo, the intent-to-treat analysis failed to show a significant difference between the groups (Ninan et al., 2000).

In a 7-week open-label trial (Koran et al., 2002), 17 of 24 subjects with CS (71%) responded to citalopram. In a subsequent study, 24 subjects received 7 weeks of open-label citalopram; 15 subjects (63%) were considered responders and entered into a double-blind phase in which they were randomly assigned to 9 weeks of treatment with citalopram or placebo (Koran et al., 2003). Compulsive shopping symptoms returned in 5 of 8 subjects (62.5%) assigned to placebo compared to none of the 7 who continued taking citalopram. Surprisingly, in an identically designed discontinuation trial by the same investigators (Koran et al., 2007), escitalopram did not separate from placebo. In this study, 19 of 26 women (73%) responded to open-label escitalopram, and 17 were then randomized to further treatment with the drug or placebo. At the end of the 9-week double-blind phase, 5 of 8 (62.5%) escitalopram recipients had relapsed, compared to 6 of 9 (66.7%) placebo recipients.

Grant (2003) and Kim (1998) described cases in which individuals with CS improved with naltrexone treatment, suggesting that opiate antagonists may have a role in the treatment of CS. Grant et al. (2012) used memantine, an N-methyl-D-aspartate receptor antagonist that may reduce glutamate excitability, in nine people with CS and reported that eight had "much" or "very much" improvement.

Whereas open-label medication trials have generally produced positive results in CS, controlled trials have not. Interpretation of these study results is complicated by placebo response rates as high as 64% (Black et al., 2000). Because the drug treatment study findings are mixed, no empirically well-supported treatment recommendations can be made.

Self-help books include *Shopaholics: Serious Help for Addicted Spenders* (Damon, 1988), *Born to Spend: How to Overcome Compulsive Spending* (Arenson, 1991), *Women Who Shop Too Much: Overcoming the Urge to Splurge* (Wesson, 1991), *Consuming Passions: Help for Compulsive Shoppers* (Catalano and Sonenberg, 1993), *Addicted to Shopping . . . and Other Issues Women Have With Money* (O'Connor, 2005), and *To Buy or Not to Buy: Why We Overshop and How to Stop* (Benson, 2008). Each provides sensible recommendations that individuals can implement to help gain control over their inappropriate shopping and spending.

Debtors Anonymous, patterned after Alcoholics Anonymous, may also be helpful (Levine and Kellen, 2000). This voluntary group provides an atmosphere of mutual support and encouragement for those with substantial debts. Simplicity circles are available in some U.S. cities; these voluntary groups encourage people to adopt a simple lifestyle and to abandon their CS (Andrews, 2000). Marriage (or couples) counseling may be helpful, particularly when CS in one member of the dyad is disrupting the relationship (Mellan, 2000). Many individuals with CS develop financial difficulties and can benefit from financial recovery counseling (McCall, 2000). The author has seen cases in which appointing a financial conservator to control the patient's finances has been helpful. Although a conservator controls the patient's spending, this approach does not reverse the individual's preoccupation with shopping.

FUTURE DIRECTIONS

Research during the past 25 years has contributed to a greater understanding of CS and its epidemiology, phenomenology, family history, etiology, and treatment. The disorder is common and is associated with comorbid psychiatric disorders; CS can lead to serious functional impairment, financial problems, and legal entanglements. More work is needed to better understand the disorder.

First, although several definitions have been proposed, most prominently the criteria of McElroy et al. (1994), their reliability and validity have not been established. Second, the issue of gender differences has been poorly studied, although it appears to be a female preponderant disorder. The survey by Koran et al. (2006) suggests that CS affects men and women equally, but this conclusion is at odds with other surveys, as well as nearly all clinical data. Gender and other risk factors require additional study.

Third, CS may be chronic or intermittent, but two studies suggest that its course may be modified with treatment. Treatment studies suggest that CBT methods may be useful, but medication studies have been inconsistent and bedeviled by high placebo response rates. More work is needed to show the superiority of medication over placebo. Follow-up studies would be helpful in charting the course of the disorder, tracking its emergence or subsidence, and confirming its relationship with other psychiatric disorders.

Finally, whether CS represents a single construct or has multiple subtypes each with its own etiologies or pathophysiology is just beginning to be explored. The classification of CS remains unclear, and research has linked it to substance use, mood, obsessive–compulsive, and impulse control disorders. Neurobiological and genetic studies would help clarify these links. As the field moves forward, more research along these domains may ultimately result in its inclusion as a formal psychiatric diagnosis, under the rubric of either substance use and related addictions or impulse control disorders more broadly.

REFERENCES

Aboujaoude, E., Gamel, N., Koran, L.M., 2003. A 1-year naturalistic follow-up of patients with compulsive shopping disorder. J Clin Psychiatry. 64, 946–950.

American Psychiatric Association, 2013. *Diagnostic and statistical manual of mental disorders* (5th ed.). Washington, DC: American Psychiatric Association.

Andrews, C., 2000. Simplicity circles and the compulsive shopper. In: Benson, A. (Ed.), I shop, therefore I am—Compulsive buying and the search for self (pp. 484–496). New York, Aronson.

Arenson, G., 1991. Born to spend: How to overcome compulsive spending. Blue Ridge Summit, PA: Tab Books.

Baker, J.H., 1987. Mary Todd Lincoln—A biography. New York: Norton.

Barratt, E., 1959. Anxiety and impulsiveness related to psychomotor efficiency. Percept Motor Skills. 9, 191–198.

Benson, A., 2008. To buy or not to buy: Why we overshop and how to stop. New York: Trumpetter.

Benson, A., Gengler, M., 2004. Treating compulsive buying. In: Coombs, R. (Ed.), Addictive disorders: A practical handbook (pp. 451–491). New York: Wiley.

Benson, A.L., Eisenach, D., Abrams, L., Van Stolk-Cooke, K., 2014. Stopping Overshopping: a preliminary randomized controlled trial of group therapy for compulsive buying disorder. J Groups Addictions Recovery. 9, 97–125.

Bernik, M.A., Akerman, D., Amaral, J.A.M.S., Braun, R.C.D.N., 1996. Cue exposure in compulsive buying (letter). J Clin Psychiatry. 57, 90.

Black, D.W., 2001. Compulsive buying disorder: Definition, assessment, epidemiology and clinical management. CNS Drugs. 15, 17–27.

Black, D.W., Monahan, P., Gabel, J., 1997. Fluvoxamine in the treatment of compulsive buying. J Clin Psychiatry. 58, 159–163.

Black, D.W., Repertinger, S., Gaffney, G. R., Gabel, J., 1998. Family history and psychiatric comorbidity in persons with compulsive buying: Preliminary findings. Am J Psychiatry. 155, 960–963.

Black, D.W., Gabel, J., Hansen, J., Schlosser, S., 2000. A double-blind comparison of fluvoxamine versus placebo in the treatment of compulsive buying disorders. Ann Clin Psychiatry. 12, 205–211.

Black, D.W., Monahan, P., Schlosser, S., Repertinger, S., 2001. Compulsive buying severity: An analysis of Compulsive Buying Scale results in 44 subjects. J Nerv Ment Dis. 189, 123–127.

Black, D.W., Shaw, M., McCormick, B., Bayless, J., Allen, J., 2012. Neuropsychological performance, impulsivity, symptoms of ADHD, and novelty seeking in compulsive buying disorder. Psychiatry Res. 200, 581–587.

Black, D.W., Coryell, W.H., Crowe, R.R., Shaw, M., McCormick, B., Allen, J. 2015. The relationship of DSM-IV pathological gambling to compulsive buying and other possible spectrum disorders: results from the Iowa PG family study. Psychiatry Res. Jan 13 [Epub ahead of print].

Bleuler, E., 1930. Textbook of psychiatry (A.A. Brill, Trans.). New York: Macmillan.

Burgard, M., Mitchell, J.E., 2000. Group cognitive–behavioral therapy for buying disorders. In: Benson, A. (Ed.), I shop, therefore I am: Compulsive buying and the search for self (pp. 367–397). New York: Aronson.

Castelot, A., 1957. Queen of France—A biography of Marie Antoinette. New York: Harper & Brothers.

Catalano, E.M., Sonenberg, N., 1993. Consuming passions—Help for compulsive shoppers. Oakland, CA: New Harbinger.

Christenson, G.A., Faber, J.R., de Zwann, M., Raymond, N.C., Specker, S.M., Ekern, M.D., et al., 1994. Compulsive buying: Descriptive characteristics and psychiatric comorbidity. J Clin Psychiatry. 55, 5–11.

Comings, D.E., Gade, R., Wu, S., Chiu, C., Dietz, G., Muhleman, D., et al.,1997. Studies of the potential role of the dopamine D1 receptor gene in addictive behaviors. Mol Psychiatry. 2, 44–56.

Damon, J.E., 1988. Shopaholics: Serious help for addicted spenders. Los Angeles: Price Stein Sloan.

Derbyshire, K., Chamberlain, S.R., Odlaug, B.L., Schreiber, L.R.N., Grant, J.E., 2014. Neurocognitive functioning in compulsive buying disorder. Ann Clin Psychiatry. 26, 57–63.

DeSarbo, W.S., Edwards, E.A., 1996. Typologies of compulsive buying behavior: A constrained clusterwise regression approach. J Consum Psychol. 5, 231–262.

Devor, E.J., Magee, H.J., Dill-Devor, R.M., Gabel, J., Black, D.W., 1999. Serotonin transporter gene (5-HTT) polymorphisms and compulsive buying. Am J Med Genet. 88, 123–125.

Di Nicola, M., Tedeschi, D., Mazza, M., Martinotti, G., Harnic, D., Catalano, V., et al.,2010. Behavioural addictions in bipolar disorder patients: Role of impulsivity and personality dimensions. J Affect Disord. 125, 82–88.

Dittmar, H., 2004. Understanding and diagnosing compulsive buying. In: Coombs, R. (Ed.), Addictive disorders: A practical handbook (pp. 411–450). New York, Wiley.

Dittmar, H., 2005. Compulsive buying—A growing concern? An examination of gender, age, and endorsement of materialistic values as predictors. Br J Psychol. 96, 467–491.

Dittmar, H., 2007. When a better self is only a button click away: Associations between materialistic values, emotional and identity-related buying motives, and compulsive buying tendency online. J Soc Clin Psychol. 26, 334–361.

Dittmar, H., Drury, J., 2000. Self-image—Is it in the bag? A qualitative comparison between "ordinary" and "excessive" consumers. J Econ Psychol. 21, 109–142.

du Toit, P.L., van Kradenburg, J., Niehaus, D., Stein, D.J., 2001. Comparison of obsessive–compulsive disorder patients with and without comorbid putative obsessive–compulsive spectrum disorders using a structured clinical interview. Compr Psychiatry. 42, 291–300.

Edwards, E.A., 1993. Development of a new scale to measure compulsive buying behavior. Fin Counsel Plan. 4, 67–84.

Elliott, R., 1994. Addictive consumption: Function and fragmentation in postmodernity. J Consum Policy. 17, 159–179.

Elliott, R., Eccles, S., Gournay, K., 1996. Revenge, existential choice, and addictive consumption. Psychol Marketing. 13, 753–768.

Erickson, C., 1991. To the scaffold—The life of Marie Antoinette. New York: Morrow.

Faber, R.J., 1992. Money changes everything: Compulsive buying from a biopsychosocial perspective. Am Behav Sci. 35, 809–819.

Faber, R.J., Christenson, G.A., 1996. In the mood to buy: Differences in the mood states experienced by compulsive buyers and other consumers. Psychol Marketing. 13, 803–820.

Faber, R.J., O'Guinn, T.C., 1989. Classifying compulsive consumers: Advances in the development of a diagnostic tool. Adv Consum Res. 16, 147–157.

Faber, R.J., O'Guinn, T.C., 1992. A clinical screener for compulsive buying. J Consum Res. 19, 459–469.

Farrell, J., 2003. One nation under goods: Malls and the seduction of the American shopper. Washington, DC: Smithsonian.

Frost, R.O., Kim, H.J., Morris, C., Bloss, C., Murray-Close, M., Steketee, G., 1998. Hoarding, compulsive buying and reasons for saving. Behav Res Ther. 36, 657–664.

Frost, R.O., Meagher, B.M., Riskind, J.H., 2001. Obsessive–compulsive features in pathological lottery and scratch-ticket gamblers. J Gamb Stud. 17, 5–19.

Glatt, M.M., Cook, C.C., 1987. Pathological spending as a form of psychological dependence. Br J Addiction. 82, 1252–1258.

Goldman, R., 2000. Compulsive buying as an addiction. In: Benson, A. (Ed.), I shop, therefore I am: Compulsive buying and the search for self (pp. 245–267). New York: Aronson.

Goodman, W.K., Price, L.H., Rasmussen. S.A., Mazure, C., Delgado, P., Heninger, G.R., et al., 1989. The Yale–Brown Obsessive–Compulsive Scale: II. Validity. Arch Gen Psychiatry. 46, 1012–1016.

Grant, J.E., 2003. Three cases of compulsive buying treated with naltrexone. Int J Psychiatry Clin Pract. 7, 223–225.

Grant, J.E., Levine, L., Kim, D., Potenza, M.N., 2005. Impulse control disorders in adult psychiatric inpatients. Am J Psychiatry. 162, 2184–2188.

Grant, J.E., Odlaug, B., Mooney, M., O'Brien, R., Kim, S.W., 2012. Open-label pilot study of memantine in the treatment of compulsive buying. Ann Clin Psychiatry. 24, 119–126.

Guy, W., 1976. ECDEU Assessment Manual for Psychopharmacology. Washington, DC: U.S. Department of HEW Publication, 217–222.

Hantouche, E.G., Bourgeois, M., Bouhassira, M., Lancrenon, S., 1996. Clinical aspects of obsessive–compulsive syndromes: Results of phase 2 of a large French survey. Encephale. 22, 255–263.

Hantouche, E.G., Lancrenon, S., Bouhassira, M., Ravily, V., Bourgeois, M.L., 1997. Repeat evaluation of impulsiveness in a cohort of 155 patients with obsessive–compulsive disorder: 12 months' prospective follow-up. Encephale. 23, 83–90.

Hartson, H., 2012. The case for compulsive shopping as an addiction. J Psychoactive Drugs. 44, 64–67.

Harvanko, A., Lust, K., Odlaug, B.L., Schreiber, L.R.N., Derbyshire, K., Christenson, G., et al., 2013. Prevalence and characteristics of compulsive buying in college students. Psychiatry Res. 210, 1079–1085.

Hassay, D.N., Smith, C.L., 1996. Compulsive buying: An examination of consumption motive. Psychol Market. 13, 741–752.

Heymann, C.D., 1989. A woman named Jackie. New York: Lyle Stuart.

Holden, C., 2001. Behavioral addictions: Do they exist? Science. 294, 980–982.

Hollander, E. (Ed.), 1993. Obsessive–compulsive related disorders. Washington, DC: American Psychiatric Press.

Hollander, E., Allen, A., 2006. Is compulsive buying a real disorder, and is it really compulsive? Am J Psychiatry. 163, 1670–1672.

Kim, S.W., 1998. Opioid antagonists in the treatment of impulse-control disorders. J Clin Psychiatry. 59, 159–164.

Knutson, B., Rick, S., Wimmer, G.E., Prelec, D., Loewenstein, G., 2007. Neural predictors of purchases. Neuron. 53, 147–153.

Koran, L.M., Bullock, K.D., Hartson, H.J., Elliott, M.A., D'Andrea, V., 2002. Citalopram treatment of compulsive shopping: An open-label study. J Clin Psychiatry. 63, 704–708.

Koran, L.M., Chuang, H.W., Bullock, K.D., Smith, S.C., 2003. Citalopram for compulsive shopping disorder: An open-label study followed by a double-blind discontinuation. J Clin Psychiatry. 64, 793–798.

Koran, L.M., Faber, R.J., Aboujaoude, E., Large, M.D., Serpe, R.T., 2006. Estimated prevalence of compulsive buying in the United States. Am J Psychiatry. 163, 1806–1812.

Koran, L.M., Aboujaoude, E.N., Solvason, B., Gamel, N., Smith, E.H., 2007. Escitalopram for compulsive buying disorder: A double-blind discontinuation study (letter). J Clin Psychopharmacol. 27, 225–227.

Kraepelin, E., 1915. Psychiatrie (8th ed., pp. 408–409). Leipzig: Verlag Von Johann Ambrosius Barth.

Krueger, D.W., 1988. On compulsive shopping and spending: A psychodynamic inquiry. Am J Psychother. 42, 574–584.

Krueger D.W., 2000. The use of money as an action symptom. In Benson AL (ed.): I Shop, Therefore I Am, Northvale, NJ: Jason Aronson Inc., 288–310.

Krych, R., 1989. Abnormal consumer behavior: A model of addictive behaviors. Adv Consum Res. 16, 745–748.

Kwak, H., Zinkhan, G.M., Crask, M.R., 2003. Diagnostic screener for compulsive buying: Applications to the USA and South Korea. J Consum Affairs. 37, 161–169.

Kyrios, M., Steketee, G., Frost, R.O., Oh, S., 2002. Cognitions in compulsive hoarding. In: Frost, R.O., Steketee, G. (Eds.), Cognitive approaches to obsessions and compulsions: Theory, assessment, and treatment (pp. 269–289). Oxford: Elsevier.

Lawrence, L., 1990. The psychodynamics of the compulsive female shopper. Am J Psychoanal. 50, 67–70.

Lee, S., Mysyk, A., 2004. The medicalization of compulsive buying. Soc Sci Med. 58, 1709–1718.

Lejoyeux, M., Hourtane, M., Ades, J., 1995. Compulsive buying and depression (letter). J Clin Psychiatry. 56, 38.

Lejoyeux, M., Andes, J., Tassian, V., Solomon, J., 1996. Phenomenology and psychopathology of uncontrolled buying. Am J Psychiatry. 152, 1524–1529.

Lejoyeux, M., Tassian, V., Solomon, J., Ades, J., 1997. Study of compulsive buying in depressed persons. J Clin Psychiatry. 58, 169–173.

Levine, B., Kellen, B., 2000. Debtors Anonymous and psychotherapy. In: Benson, A. (Ed.), I shop, therefore I am: Compulsive buying and the search for self (pp. 431–454). New York: Jason Aronson.

Lo, H.Y., Harvey, N., 2011. Shopping without pain: Compulsive buying and the effects of credit card availability in Europe and the Far East. J Econ Psychol. 32, 79–91.

Magee, A., 1994. Compulsive buying tendency as a predictor of attitudes and perceptions. Adv Consum Res. 21, 590–594.

McCall, K., 2000. Financial recovery counseling. In: Benson, A. (Ed.), I shop, therefore I am: Compulsive buying and the search for self (pp. 457–483). New York: Aronson.

McElroy, S., Satlin, A., Pope, H.G., Jr., Keck, P.E., Hudson, J.I., 1991. Treatment of compulsive shopping with antidepressants: A report of three cases. Ann Clin Psychiatry. 3, 199–204.

McElroy, S., Keck, P.E., Pope, H.G., Jr., Smith, J.M.R., Strakowski, S.M., 1994. Compulsive buying: A report of 20 cases. J Clin Psychiatry. 55, 242–248.

Mellan, O., 2000. Overcoming overspending in couples. In: Benson, A. (Ed.), I shop, therefore I am: Compulsive buying and the search for self (pp. 341–366). New York: Aronson.

Miltenberger, R.G., Redlin, J., Crosby, R., Stickney, M., Mitchell, J., Wonderlich, S., et al., 2003. Direct and retrospective assessment of factors contributing to compulsive buying. J Behav Ther Experiment Psychiatry. 34, 1–9.

Mitchell, J.E., Burgard, M., Faber, R., Crosby, R.D., 2006. Cognitive behavioral therapy for compulsive buying disorder. Behav Res Ther. 44, 1859–1865.

Monahan, P., Black, D.W., Gabel, J., 1996. Reliability and validity of a scale to measure change in persons with compulsive buying. Psychiatry Res. 64, 59–67.

Mueller, A., Mitchell, J.E., Mertens, C., Mueller, U., Silbermann, A., Burgard, M., et al., 2007. Comparison of treatment seeking compulsive buyers in Germany and the United States. Behav Res Ther. 45, 1629–1638.

Mueller, A., Mueller, U., Silbermann, A., Reinecker, H., Bleich, S., Mitchell, J.E., et al., 2008. A randomized, controlled trial of group cognitive behavioral therapy for compulsive buying disorder: Posttreatment and 6-month follow-up results. J Clin Psychiatry. 69, 1131–1138.

Mueller, A., Mühlhans, B., Müller, U., Mertens, C., Horbach, T., Michell, J.E., et al., 2009. Compulsive buying and psychiatric comorbidity. Psychother Psychosom Med Psychol. 59, 291–299.

Mueller, A., Mitchell, J.E., Black, D.W., Crosby, R.D., Berg, K., De Zwaan, M., 2010. Latent profile analysis and comorbidity in a sample of individuals with compulsive buying disorder. Biol Psychiatry. 178, 348–353.

Muller, A., Mitchell, J.E., de Zwaan, M., 2013. Compulsive buying. Am J Addictions. 24(2), 132–137.

Murphy, D.L., Pickar, D.L., Alterman, I.S., 1982. Methods or the quantitative assessment of depressive and manic behavior. In: Burdock, E.I., Sudilovski, A., & Gershon, S. (Eds.), The Behavior of Psychiatric Patients. New York: Marcel Dekker, 355–391.

Nataraajan, R., Goff, B.G., 1991. Compulsive buying: Toward a reconceptualization. J Soc Behav Personality. 6, 307–328.

Neuner, M., Raab, G., Reisch, L., 2005. Compulsive buying in maturing consumer societies: An empirical re-inquiry. J Econ Psychol. 26, 509–522.

Ninan, P.T., McElroy, S.L., Kane, C.P., Knight, B.T., Casuto, L.S., Rose, S.E., et al., 2000. Placebo-controlled study of fluvoxamine in the treatment of patients with compulsive buying. J Clin Psychopharmacol. 20, 362–366.

O'Connor, K., 2005. Addicted to shopping ... and other issues women have with money. Eugene, OR: Harvest House.

O'Guinn, T.C., Faber, R.J., 1989. Compulsive buying: A phenomenological exploration. J Consum Res. 16, 147–157.

Otero-Lopez, J.M., Pol, E.V., 2013. Compulsive buying and the Five Factor model of personality: A facet analysis. Person Ind Differences. 55, 585–590.

Otter, M., Black, D.W., 2007. Compulsive buying behavior in two mentally challenged persons. Primary Care Companion J Clin Psychiatry. 9, 469–470.

Raab, G., Reisch, L., Gwozdz, W., Kollman, K., Schubert, A.M., Unger, A., 2012. Pathological buying behavior: Investigating the trend of compensatory and compulsive buying in Austria, Denmark, and Germany. In: Gasiorowska, A., Zaleskiewicz, T. (Eds.), Microcosm of economic psychology: Proceedings of the IAREP Conference Wroclaw 2012. Wroclaw: Warsaw School of Social Sciences and Humanities Faculty.

Richards, A.K., 1996. Ladies of fashion: Pleasure, perversion or paraphilia. Int J Psychoanal. 77, 337–351.

Ridgeway, N.M., Kukar-Kinney, M., Monroe, K.B., 2008. An expanded conceptualization and a new measure of compulsive buying. J Consum Res. 35, 350–406.

Roberts, J.A., 1998. Compulsive buying among college students: An investigation of its antecedents, consequences, and implications for public policy. J Consum Affairs, 32, 295–319.

Roberts, J.A., Sepulveda, C.J., 1999. Money attitudes and compulsive buying: An exploratory investigation of the emerging consumer culture in Mexico. J Int Consum Market. 11, 53–74.

Roberts, J.A., Tanner, J.F., Jr., 2000. Compulsive buying and risky behavior among adolescents. Psychol Rep. 86, 763–770.

Roberts, J.A., Tanner, J.F., Jr., 2002. Compulsive buying and sexual attitudes, intentions, and activity among adolescents: An extension of Roberts and Tanner. Psychol Rep. 90, 1259–1260.

Scherhorn, G., Reisch, L.A., Raab, G., 1990. Addictive buying in West Germany: An empirical study. J Consum Policy. 13, 355–387.

Schlosser, S., Black, D.W., Repertinger, S., Freet, D., 1994. Compulsive buying: Demography, phenomenology, and comorbidity in 46 subjects. Gen Hosp Psychiatry. 16, 205–212.

Schwartz, H.J., 1992. Psychoanalytic psychotherapy for a woman with diagnoses of kleptomania and bulimia. Hosp Com Psychiatry. 43, 109–110.

Stekel, W., 1924. Peculiarities of behavior (J. S. Van Teslaar, Trans.). New York: Liveright.

Swanberg, W.A., 1961. Citizen hearst. New York: Galahad.

Valence, G., d'Astous, A., Fortier, L., 1988. Compulsive buying: Concept and measurement. J Clin Policy. 11, 419–433.

Villarino, R., Otero-Lopez, J.L., Casto, R., 2001. Adicion a la compra: Analysis, evaluaction y tratamiento [Buying addiction: Analysis, evaluation, and treatment]. Madrid: Ediciones Piramide.

Villella, C., Martinotti, G., Di Nicola, M., Cassano, M., La Torre, G., Gliubizzi, M.D., et al., 2011. Behavioral addictions in adolescents and young adults: Results from a prevalence study. J Gamb Stud. 27, 203–214.

Wesson, C., 1991. Women who shop too much: Overcoming the urge to splurge. New York: St. Martin's Press.

Weun, S., Jones, M.A., Beatty, S.E., 1998. Development and validation of the Impulse Buying Tendency Scale. Psychol Rep. 82, 1123–1133.

Winestine, M.C.,1985. Compulsive shopping as a derivative of childhood seduction. Psychoanal Q. 54, 70–72.

World Health Organization, 2007. International classification of diseases (10th ed.). Geneva: World Health Organization.

Yurchistan, J., Johnson, K.K.P., 2007. Compulsive buying behavior and its relationship to perceived social status associated with buying, materialism, self esteem, and apparel product involvement. Family Consum Sci Res J. 32, 291–314.

Zuckerman, M., 1994. Behavioral expressions and biosocial bases of sensation seeking. New York: Cambridge University Press.

7

Exercise Addiction

*Diagnosis, Psychobiological Mechanisms,
and Treatment*

AVIV WEINSTEIN AND YITZHAK WEINSTEIN ■

Exercise and physical activity are beneficial both physiologically and psychologically (Bouchard et al., 1994), but some individuals may engage in exercise excessively, resulting in physical as well as psychological damage. It has been argued that excessive exercise may be harmful or addictive (Szabo, 1995, 1998, 2000; Yates, 1991).

Exercising to excess has been described within both an addiction framework (i.e., exercise addiction) and an obsessive–compulsive spectrum (Demetrovics and Kurimay, 2008). Some excessive exercisers appear to experience powerful withdrawal symptoms (Szabo, 1995) along with physical, medical, financial, and social problems that parallel those of other addictions (for review, see Berczik et al., 2012). This chapter summarizes the phenomenology of exercise addiction, with emphasis on the physiological and neuropharmacological mechanisms responsible for its rewarding and addictive properties. In line with Berczik et al., the term "exercise addiction" is used throughout the chapter because addictions incorporate both dependence and compulsive features, which appear to apply to excessive exercising as well as to other behavioral addictions.

DEFINING FEATURES AND METHODS FOR ASSESSMENT

Although exercise addition is not included in the fifth edition of the *Diagnostic and Statistical Manual of Mental Disorders* (DSM-5; American Psychiatric Association, 2013), parallels are often made with other behavioral addictions, such as substance use disorders and gambling disorder. For example, Griffiths (1996, 1997, 2002, 2005) suggested that exercise addiction may share features of other addictions, namely salience, mood modification, tolerance, withdrawal symptoms, conflict between the individual and his or her peers, and reductions in other activities. Relapse, referring to the tendency to return to excessive activity after periods of abstinence or control, has also been reported (Berczik et al., 2012). Morgan (1979) suggested that exercise addiction can have detrimental psychological and social consequences and interfere with relationships and work as well. Several studies have reported that when prevented from exercising, addicted exercisers experience withdrawal symptoms, including depression, irritability, and anxiety (Adams and Kirby, 2002; Aidman and Woollard, 2003; Allegre et al., 2006). Szabo (1995) suggested that people who exercise regularly do so to cope with stress. Although these preliminary studies suggest some similarities between symptoms of exercise addiction and substance use disorders, it is not yet clear how best to define or assess exercise addiction.

Currently, there are no common methods for assessing excessive exercising, but several instruments have been developed. The Obligatory Exercise Questionnaire (OEQ) (Ackard et al., 2002) includes 20 items and covers a wide range of exercise behaviors and cognitions, such as frequency of exercising and fixation on and commitment to exercising. The Exercise Dependence Questionnaire (EDQ) (Ogden et al., 1997) consists of 29 items investigating the social effects and motivational factors of exercise, including reward and withdrawal symptoms. The Exercise Dependence Scale (EDS) (Hausenblas and Symons Downs, 2002) was founded on the DSM-IV criteria for substance dependence and assesses similar symptoms such as withdrawal, tolerance, and lack of control (American Psychiatric Association, 1994) with 21 items. It also assesses craving for exercise, which parallels a criterion of substance use disorders in DSM-5. The OEQ has acceptable internal consistency, and it is correlated with EDS scores (Hausenblas and Symons Downs, 2002).

The Exercise Addiction Inventory (EAI) is a short questionnaire with six items, assessing salience, mood changes, tolerance, withdrawal, conflict, and relapse. The EAI has a high correlation with the EDS (Griffiths et al., 2005; Terry et al., 2004) and the EDQ (Monok et al., 2012). An instrument developed specifically for runners, the Running Addiction Scale (Chapman and De Castro, 1990) has shown that self-reports of high-frequency running are related to commitment to run, whereas duration of running is related to mood enhancement effects.

As noted previously, many instruments exist to address aspects of exercise addiction, and some are highly correlated. However, none are standardly applied, and the defining features and adverse consequences of exercise addition are not well-established. Thus, more research is necessary to define and assess this condition before excessive exercising can be considered a mental disorder and before recommendations can be made regarding whether this condition is best aligned with addictive disorders or other psychiatric conditions.

PREVALENCE RATES

Prevalence rates of exercise addiction are described in Table 7.1. The top section of the table reports prevalence rates from subsets of the general population that is not limited to athletes—that is, primarily students and persons who exercise regularly but who are not athletes per se. Studies from specific athlete populations, who are likely to have higher rates of exercise addiction than the general population, are shown in the lower section of the table.

There are relatively few studies of the prevalence of exercise addition, and existing studies span countries as well as the populations surveyed. In surveys of students, the prevalence rates range from as low as 2.5% (Terry et al., 2004) to greater than 25% (MacLaren and Best, 2010).

Table 7.1 PREVALENCE OF EXERCISE ADDICTION

Study	Country and Study Population	No. of Subjects	Prevalence Rate (%)
NOT LIMITED TO ATHLETE POPULATIONS			
Garman et al. (2004)	United States, students	257	21.8
Terry et al. (2004)	United Kingdom, students	200	2.5
Griffiths et al. (2005)	United Kingdom, exercising population	200	3
Szabo and Griffiths (2007)	United Kingdom, university sports science students	261	6.9
Lejoyeux et al. (2008)	France, adolescent exercising population	300	42
MacLaren and Best (2010)	Canada, students	948	25.6
Villella et al. (2011)	Italy, school adolescents	2,853	8.5
Lejoyeux et al. (2012)	France, sports shop customers	500	29.6
ATHLETE POPULATIONS			
Blaydon and Lindner (2002)	Hong Kong, triathletes	203	30.4
Allegre et al. (2007)	UK, ultra marathoners	95	3.2
McNamara and McCabe (2012)	Australia, elite athletes	234	34

Clearly, individuals who do not exercise cannot be addicted to exercising, and some studies have restricted assessment to those who report they do exercise. Rates of exercise addiction in exercising populations have also varied vastly from as low as 3% (Griffiths et al., 2005) to up to 42% (Lejoyeux et al., 2008). A variety of instruments were applied across these studies, as well as different methods for scoring and classifying addiction to exercise. Given these discrepancies, the prevalence rates of this condition are not well understood.

The lower section of Table 7.1 shows studies assessing exercise addiction among athlete samples specifically. The prevalence rates of exercise addiction in athletes is reported to be as high as 30.4% among triathletes

(Blaydon and Lindner, 2002) and 25% among runners (Slay et al., 1998) to as low as 3.2% among "ultra-marathoners" (Allegre et al., 2007). Again, the different rates across samples likely reflect use of different assessment instruments, as well as different sampling techniques. In addition, it is possible that persons more prone to developing problems with exercise may gravitate more toward certain sports. As demonstrated in Table 7.1, the field lacks a good understanding of the rates of problems with exercising that develop in general populations or in specific athlete samples.

COMORBIDITIES WITH OTHER PSYCHIATRIC DISORDERS

Although exercise addiction itself is not well defined, some evidence suggests that individuals who develop problems related to exercising also suffer from other psychiatric conditions at high rates. The psychiatric condition that has most often been assessed in conjunction with exercise addition is eating disorders. Some reports (O'Dea and Abraham, 2002; Sussman et al., 2011) suggest that exercise addiction has symptoms in common and high comorbidity with eating and body image disorders. Some individuals with exercise addiction are preoccupied with their body image, and some data suggest they tend to weigh themselves regularly and exercise under dietary control (Blaydon and Lindner, 2002; Klein et al., 2004; Lyons and Cromey, 1989; Sundgot-Borgen, 1993). In one study of women, exercise addiction occurred only when an eating disorder was also present (Bamber et al., 2000). However, other studies have not found this association. Blumenthal et al. (1984) and Coen and Ogles (1993) failed to find relationships between exercise addiction and eating disorders, and in a review of the literature, Szabo (2010) could not identify conclusive evidence for a relationship between exercise addiction and eating disorders.

There is a large body of literature addressing the relationships between exercise as an activity (but not exercise addiction) and depression and anxiety. Cooney et al. (2013) reviewed 39 trials involving 2,326 people diagnosed with depression and noted moderately lower rates of depression among those who exercised relative to those who did not. Da Silva et al. (2012) reported that physical exercise can reduce anxiety and depression symptoms, whereas a lack of exercise is associated with higher levels of anxiety and depression. Exercise and regular activity are inversely associated with manifestations of anxiety symptoms in animal models as well (Da Silva et al., 2012), and numerous studies demonstrate that higher levels of exercise activities are related to reduced levels of anxiety in clinical samples (Anderson and Shivakumar, 2013). However, there are very few studies that directly address the association between exercise addiction and depression and anxiety symptoms.

Although exercise addiction has been assumed to share features with substance use and behavioral addictions, few studies have addressed the comorbidities of these disorders. In one of the few such studies, Lejoyeux et al. (2008) assessed 300 adolescents in a French fitness center. The participants completed measures of exercise addiction, alcohol and nicotine use disorders, other putative behavioral addictions such as compulsive buying and Internet addiction, and two disorders related to anxiety focused on the body—bulimia and hypochondria. In the full sample, 125 subjects (42%) were classified with exercise addiction. Unsurprisingly, these individuals spent more hours each day in the fitness center than individuals who were not classified with exercise addiction (2.1 vs. 1.5 hours per day, respectively). They also went to the fitness center more often each week (3.5 vs. 2.9 days per week). Those classified with exercise addiction smoked less, but alcohol consumption was equivalent in the groups. Compulsive buying was significantly more frequent in those with exercise addiction (63% vs. 38%), and those classified with exercise addiction scored higher on a compulsive buying scale. The prevalence of hypochondria was equivalent in both groups, but scores on a scale of hypochondria were higher in the exercise addicted group. Bulimia was significantly more frequent among those with exercise addiction (70% vs. 47%). Subjects with exercise addiction spent more time on their computer each day (3.9 vs. 2.4 hours per day), and they also reported greater time on the Internet explicitly and sending and receiving more e-mail. Thus, in this sample of adolescent fitness center attendees, those classified with exercise addition appeared to evidence increased rates of some other excessive behavioral patterns, such as shopping and Internet use, but they smoked less and had equivalent rates of alcohol use.

In summary, there are very few studies assessing the co-occurrence of exercise addiction with other Axis I disorders, such as mood, anxiety, or substance use disorders. Exercise addiction may be related to eating disorders, but even data on this association are mixed. There is a need for further research related to the prevalence of exercise addiction, as well as its association with other psychiatric conditions to understand whether it aligns best with behavioral addictions or other conditions.

RISK AND PROTECTIVE FACTORS

Several risk factors for developing exercise addiction have been proposed, including demographics and personality characteristics, as well as some biological and genetic predispositions.

Gender has been explored as a possible risk factor for exercise addiction (for review, see Fattore et al., 2014). Initially, Pierce et al. (1997) reported that women marathon runners had significantly higher exercise addiction scores than men. These findings were confirmed by Hausenblas and Symons Downs (2002) in a study of 408 university students, as well as by Blaydon and Lindner (2002). Weik and Hale (2009) likewise found that male exercisers had significantly higher total EDS scores than females, but Zmijewski and Howard (2003) noted that women more often reported craving for exercise and being nervous when unable to exercise. However, other studies showed no sex differences in "addiction" to running and exercising (Furst and Germone 1993; Greenberg et al., 1999).

Personality may be a risk factor for engaging in adventurous sport that may be addictive (Cloninger et al., 1993). The personality traits of high novelty seeking and low harm avoidance are related to drug abuse, as well as participation in adventurous sports (Ebstein et al., 1996). Molecular genetic studies find associations between the dopamine *DRD4* exon III repeat region and novelty seeking/extraversion and with the serotonin transporter (*SLC6A4*) promoter region polymorphism (*5-HTTLPR*) and neuroticism/harm avoidance (Ebstein et al., 1996). Although these genes have been studied widely in the context of substance use disorders, no such molecular genetic studies have been conducted with respect to exercise addiction. Future research may examine pharmacogenetic factors that may relate to the vulnerability to become addicted to adventurous sports.

Genetic studies also suggest that the same genes that impact preference for drugs may play a role in preference for other naturally rewarding behaviors such as exercise (Brené et al., 2007). For example, dopamine may contribute to excessive exercise activities such as wheel running in mice. Greater dopamine concentrations were noted in the dorsal striatum and nucleus accumbens of high wheel running mice compared with mice bred for obesity and a nonselected strain (Mathes et al., 2010). Furthermore, wheel running is rewarding, as measured by conditioned place preference and increased immune reactivity in the nucleus accumbens in rats (Greenwood et al., 2011). Genetic or environmental alterations that impact central reward pathways may contribute to exercise addiction, although these relationships have not been well studied in humans.

Relatedly, exercise is known to induce the "runner's high," an analgesic and euphoric mental state. The "endorphin hypothesis of exercise" suggests that exercise-induced changes in psychological functions are a direct consequence of alterations in endogenous opioid release (Thompson and Blanton, 1987). Using brain imaging techniques, Boecker et al. (2008) examined opioid release with a nonselective opioid ligand and found that athletes who were scanned after 2 hours of endurance running evidenced reduced opioid receptor availability in the prefrontal and the limbic/para limbic brain structures. Ratings of euphoria were significantly increased after running, and they were inversely correlated with opioid binding in prefrontal/orbitofrontal cortices, the anterior cingulate cortex, bilateral insula, parainsular cortex, and temporal–parietal regions. These findings suggest region-specific effects in frontal–limbic brain areas that are involved in the processing of affective states and mood and may relate to exercise addiction. In addition, the endocannabinoid system has been reported to be associated with runner's high, potentially relating to addictive properties as well (Dietrich and McDaniel, 2004). The close interaction of endocannabinoids with opioids and dopamine suggests they may work together in the reward system related to multiple addictions, including that associated with exercise, but these hypotheses require further investigation.

TREATMENTS

Treatment approaches for exercise addiction are often based on motivational and cognitive–behavioral approaches, similar to those used in the treatment of substance use and gambling disorders. However, there is little evidence on the effectiveness of interventions for exercise addiction, and no randomized controlled trials exist.

Clinically, assessment and treatment usually takes into account the duration of exercise addiction and comorbidity with other psychiatric disorders such as eating disorders (Freimuth et al., 2011). Primary exercise addiction occurs in the absence of an eating disorder. In these cases, any weight loss is secondary to calories burned from exercising, or if there is dieting, it occurs solely for the purpose of improving performance. However, for some people, the primary motivation for excessive exercising appears to be weight loss, and in these cases, eating disorders must be addressed in the context of therapy as well.

One of the first issues in treatment, whether exercise addiction is primary or secondary, is to motivate patients to remain in therapy, given that many are insufficiently aware of the adverse effects generated by their behavior. Once motivated and engaged in treatment, attention can turn to identifying and correcting automatic and erroneous thoughts related to exercise. These may include those related to desiring to control body image and also the idea that exercise is always good even if it is performed in an obsessive manner. Second, when treating exercise addiction, abstinence from exercise may not be the desired goal because exercise in moderation is considered a healthy habit. A typical treatment goal is to return to moderate levels of exercise. In some cases, a new form of exercise may be recommended—for example, the runner is encouraged to swim or cycle. In other cases, the person may continue to do the same form of exercise in a more controlled or less intensive manner. Whether moderating the original exercise behavior or replacing one activity with another, clinicians should assist patients in distinguishing problematic or addictive exercise from moderate or recreational exercise (Freimuth et al., 2011).

Only a single case study is available on potential pharmacological treatment of exercise addiction. Di Nicola et al. (2010) provided quetiapine, an antipsychotic, as an add-on treatment for a patient with bipolar I disorder and comorbid compulsive buying and exercise addiction. After 4 weeks of treatment, the patient showed mild improvement of both his buying behaviors and excessive exercise activities. After 12 weeks, more pronounced reductions in symptoms were noted, and they had resolved by 24 weeks of treatment. Scores on the EAI decreased markedly after treatment. Although this report suggests potential of this medication, it represents a single case study of a patient with multiple disorders. Clearly, more and rigorously controlled studies are needed prior to drawing conclusions about either pharmacological or psychological treatments for exercise addiction.

FUTURE DIRECTIONS

Prior to classifying exercise addition as a unique mental disorder, research on the definition, diagnosis, and etiology of this condition is needed. Several tools have been developed to assess excessive exercising, and they have some evidence of reliability. However, studies of the validity of these tools are lacking, and many have been utilized only in the context of a single study. The specific criteria used to assess the condition vary across instruments, and methods to define and distinguish problematic exercising from frequent but nonharmful exercising are lacking. Exercise addiction has been considered along an obsessive–compulsive dimension as well as impulsive and rewarding one, and it may also relate closely to eating disorders, at least in some cases. Whether it is distinct from or best aligns with substance use and addictive, obsessive–compulsive, or eating disorders remains debated.

To date, relatively few studies have investigated the prevalence of exercise addiction in the general population, and they point to highly variable rates. In part, the discrepancies relate to the lack of standardized assessment instruments as well as a lack of consensus on the defining characteristics of this condition.

No randomized controlled studies of treatment for exercise addiction exist. Although cognitive–behavioral and motivational approaches are applied clinically, their effectiveness is unknown. Theories exist to describe the onset and maintenance of the condition, and physiological and biological risk factors have been proposed. A better understanding of how excessive exercising develops and impacts or is influenced by physiology may ultimately guide pharmacological approaches to treat it. As the field moves closer to defining this condition, it will be important to systematically evaluate how well interventions can both prevent and treat the adverse consequences associated with excessive exercising.

ACKNOWLEDGMENTS

The authors dedicate this chapter to the memory of their parents Israel and Neomi Weinstein.

REFERENCES

Ackard, D.M., Brehm, B.J., Steffen, J.J., 2002. Exercise and eating disorders in college-aged women: Profiling excessive exercisers. Eating Disord. 10, 31–47.

Adams, J., Kirby, R.J., 2002. Excessive exercise as an addiction: A review. Addiction Res Theory. 30, 415–437.

Aidman, A.V., Woollard, S., 2003. The influence of self-reported exercise addiction on acute emotional and physiological responses to brief exercise deprivation. Psychol Sport Exerc. 4, 225–236.

Allegre, B., Souville, M., Therme, P., Griffiths, M., 2006. Definitions and measures of exercise dependence. Addiction Res Theory. 14, 631–646.

Allegre, B., Therme, P., Griffiths, M.D., 2007. Individual factors and the context of physical activity in exercise dependence: A prospective study of "ultra-marathoners." Int J Mental Health Addict. 5, 233–243.

American Psychiatric Association, 1994. Diagnostic and statistical manual of mental disorders (4th ed.). Washington, DC: American Psychiatric Association.

American Psychiatric Association, 2013. *Diagnostic and statistical manual of mental disorders* (5th ed.). Washington, DC: American Psychiatric Association.

Anderson, E., Shivakumar, G., 2013. Effects of exercise and physical activity on anxiety. Front Psychiatry. 4, 1–4.

Bamber, D., Cockerill, I., Carroll D., 2000. The pathological status of exercise dependence. Br J Sports Med. 34, 125–132.

Berczik, K., Szabó, A., Griffiths, M.D., Kurimay, T., Kun, B., Urbán, R., et al., 2012. Exercise addiction: Symptoms, diagnosis, epidemiology, and etiology. Subst Use Misuse. 47, 403–417.

Blaydon, M.J., Lindner, K.J., 2002. Eating disorders and exercise dependence in triathletes. Eating Disord. 10, 49–60.

Blumenthal, J.A., O'Toole, L.C., Chang, J.L., 1984. Is running an analogue of anorexia nervosa? An empirical study of obligatory running and anorexia nervosa. JAMA. 252, 520–523.

Boecker, H., Sprenger, T., Spilker, M.E., Henriksen, G., Koppenhoefer, M., Wagner, K.J., et al., 2008. The runner's high: Opioidergic mechanisms in the human brain. Cereb Cortex. 18, 2523–2531.

Bouchard, C., Shephard, R.J., Stephens, T., 1994. Physical activity, fitness and health: International proceedings and consensus statement. Champaign, IL: Human Kinetics.

Brené, S., Bjørnebekk, A., Aberg, E., Mathé, A.A., Olson, L., Werme, M., 2007. Running is rewarding and antidepressive. Physiol Behav. 92, 136–140.

Chapman, C.L., De Castro, J.M., 1990. Running addiction: Measurement and associated psychological characteristics. J Sports Med Phys Fitness. 30, 283–290.

Cloninger, C.R., Svrakic, D.M., Przybeck, T.R., 1993. A psychobiological model of temperament and character. Arch Gen Psychiatry. 50, 975–990.

Coen, S.P., Ogles, B.M., 1993. Psychological characteristics of the obligatory runner: A critical examination of the anorexia analogue hypothesis. J Sport Exerc Psychol. 15, 338–354.

Cooney, G.M., Dwan, K., Greig, C.A., Lawlor, D.A., Rimer, J., Waugh, F.R., McMurdo, M., Mead. G.E., 2013. Exercise for depression. Cochrane Database Syst Rev. 9, CD004366.

Da Silva, M.A., Singh-Manoux, A., Brunner, E.J., Kaffashian, S., Shipley, M.J., Kivimaki, M., et al., 2012. Bidirectional association between physical activity and symptoms of anxiety and depression: The Whitehall II study. Eur J Epidemiol. 27, 537–546.

Demetrovics, Z., Kurimay, T., 2008. Exercise addiction: A literature review. Psychiatr Hung. 23, 129–141.

Di Nicola, M., Martinotti, G., Mazza, M., Tedeschi, D., Pozzi, G., Janiri, L., 2010. Quetiapine as add-on treatment for bipolar I disorder with comorbid compulsive buying and physical exercise addiction. Prog Neuropsychopharmacol Biol Psychiatry. 34, 713–714.

Dietrich, A., McDaniel, W., 2004. Endocannabinoids and exercise. Br J Sports Med. 38,536–541.

Ebstein, R.P., Novick, O., Umansky, R., Priel, B., Osher, Y., Blaine, D., et al., 1996. Dopamine D4 receptor (D4DR) exon III polymorphism associated with the human personality trait of novelty seeking. Nat Genet. 12, 78–80.

Fattore, L., Melis, M., Fadda, P., Fratta, W., 2014. Sex differences in addictive disorders. Front Neuroendocrinol. 35, 272–284.

Freimuth, M., Moniz, S., Kim, S.R., 2011. Clarifying exercise addiction: Differential diagnosis, co-occurring disorders, and phases of addiction. Int J Environ Res Public Health. 8, 4069–4081.

Furst, D.M., Germone, K., 1993. Negative addiction in male and female runners and exercisers. Percept. Motor Skills. 77, 192–194

Garman, J.F., Hayduk, D.M., Crider, D.A., Hodel, M.M., 2004. Occurrence of exercise dependence in a college aged population. J Am Coll Health. 52, 221–228.

Greenberg, J.L., Lewis, S.E., Dodd, D.K., 1999. Overlapping addictions and self-esteem among college men and women. Addict. Behav. 24, 565–571.

Greenwood, B.N., Foley, T.E., Le, T.V., Strong, P.V., Loughridge, A.B., Day, H.E., et al., 2011. Long term voluntary wheel running is rewarding and produces plasticity in the mesolimbic reward pathway. Behav Brain Res. 217, 354–362.

Griffiths, M.D., 1996. Behavioural addiction: An issue for everybody? J Workplace Learning. 8, 19–25.

Griffiths, M.D., 1997. Exercise addiction: A case study. Addict Res Theory. 5, 161–168.

Griffiths, M.D., 2002. Gambling and gaming addictions in adolescence. Leicester, UK: British Psychological Society.

Griffiths, M.D., 2005. A "components" model of addiction within a biopsychosocial framework. J Substance Use Treat. 10, 191–197.

Griffiths, M.D., Szabo, A., Terry, A., 2005. The Exercise Addiction Inventory: A quick and easy screening tool for health practitioners. Br J Sports Med. 39, e30.

Hausenblas, H.A., Symons Downs, D., 2002. Exercise dependence: A systematic review. Psychol Sport Exerc. 3, 89–123.

Klein, D.A., Bennett, A.S., Schebendach, J., Foltin, R.W., Devlin, M.J., Walsh, B.T., 2004. Exercise "addiction" in anorexia nervosa: Model development and pilot data. CNS Spectr. 9, 531–537.

Lejoyeux, M., Avril, M., Richoux, C., Embouazza, H., Nivoli, F., 2008. Prevalence of exercise dependence and other behavioral addictions among clients of a Parisian fitness room. Compr Psychiatry. 49, 353–358.

Lejoyeux, M., Guillot, C., Chalvin, F., Petit, A., Lequen, V., 2012. Exercise dependence among customers from a Parisian sport shop. J Behav Addict. 1, 28–34.

Lyons, H.A., Cromey, R., 1989. Compulsive jogging: Exercise dependence and associated disorder of eating. Ulster Med J. 58, 100–102.

MacLaren, V.V., Best, L.A., 2010. Multiple addictive behaviors in young adults: Student norms for the Shorter PROMIS Questionnaire. Addict Behav. 35, 252–255.

Mathes, W., Nehrenberg, D., Gordon, R., Hua, K., Garland, T., Pomp, D., 2010. Dopaminergic dysregulation in mice selectively bred for excessive exercise or obesity. Behav Brain Res. 210, 155–163.

McNamara, J., McCabe, M., 2012. Striving for success or addiction? Exercise dependence among elite Australian athletes. J Sports Sci. 30, 755–766.

Monok, K., Berczik, K., Urban, R., Szabo, A., Griffiths, M., Farkas, J., et al., 2012. Psychometric properties and concurrent validity of two exercise addiction measures: A population wide study. Psychol Sport Exerc. 13, 739–746.

Morgan, W.P., 1979. Negative addiction in runners. Phys Sportsmed. 7, 57–70.

O'Dea, J.A., Abraham, S., 2002. Eating and exercise disorders in young college men. J Am Coll Health. 50, 273–278.

Ogden, J., Veale, D., Summers, Z., 1997. The development and validation of the Exercise Dependence Questionnaire. Addict Res Theory. 5, 343–356.

Pierce, E., Rohaly, K., Fritchley, B., 1997. Sex differences on exercise dependence for men and women in a marathon road race. Percept Motor Skills. 84, 991–994.

Slay, H.A., Hayaki, J., Napolitano, M.A., Brownell, K.D., 1998. Motivations for running and eating attitudes in obligatory versus nonobligatory runners. Int J Eat Disord. 23, 267–275.

Sundgot-Borgen, J., 1993. Prevalence of eating disorders in elite female athletes. Int J Sport Nutr. 3, 29–40.

Sussman, S., Lisha, N., Griffiths, M.D., 2011. Prevalence of the addictions: A problem of the majority or the minority? Eval Health Prof. 34, 3–56.

Szabo, A., 1995. The impact of exercise deprivation on well-being of habitual exercisers. Australian J Sci Med Sport. 27, 68–75.

Szabo, A., 1998. Studying the psychological impact of exercise deprivation: Are experimental studies hopeless? J Sport Behav. 21, 139–147.

Szabo, A., 2000. Physical activity and psychological dysfunction. In: Biddle, S., Fox, K. Boutcher, S. (Eds.), Physical activity and psychological well-being (pp. 130–153). London: Routledge.

Szabo, A. (2010). Addiction to exercise: A symptom or a disorder? New York: Nova Science.

Szabo, A., Griffiths, M.D., 2007. Exercise addiction in British sport science students. Int J Ment Health Addict. 5, 25–28.

Terry, A., Szabo, A., Griffiths, M., 2004. The Exercise Addiction Inventory: A new brief screening tool. Addict Res Ther. 12, 489–499.

Thompson, J.K., Blanton, P., 1987. Energy conservation and exercise dependence: A sympathetic arousal hypothesis. Med Sci Sport Exerc. 19, 91–99.

Villella, C., Martinotti, G., Di Nicola, M., Cassano, M., La Torre, G., Gliubizzi, M., et al., 2011. Behavioural addictions in adolescents and young adults: Results from a prevalence study. J Gambl Stud. 27, 203–214.

Weik, M., Hale, B.D., 2009. Contrasting gender differences on two measures of exercise dependence. Br J Sports Med. 43, 204–207.

Yates, A., 1991. Compulsive exercise and the eating disorders: Toward an integrated theory of activity. New York: Brunner/Mazel.

Zmijewski, C.F., Howard, M.O., 2003. Exercise dependence and attitudes toward eating among young adults. Eating Behav. 4, 181–195.

8

Food Addiction

SUSAN MURRAY, MARK S. GOLD,
AND NICOLE M. AVENA ■

"I tell myself I will only eat one cookie, then that leads to another and another until I make myself stop at five or six. I used to be able to eat only one or two."

—IFLAND *et al. (2009), p. 520*

"It is always a fight. Always a conflict every day. I know it is happening. I know the outcome, but I cannot stop it."

—CURTIS AND DAVIS *(2014), p. 29*

"I'm so uncomfortable after a binge.... I'm miserable ... but I overeat anyway."

—IFLAND *et al. (2009), p. 522*

Reports such as these have led some to question whether certain individuals may experience eating as an addiction. At first pass, the concept of food addiction may appear absurd given that food is needed to maintain survival; in a sense, we are all "dependent" on food. In contrast, overconsumption of highly palatable foods and cycles of food restriction coupled with overeating these kinds of foods are not necessary for survival, and these are precisely the habits that are associated with the development of addictive-like eating behavior. The subject of food addiction has been a source of inquiry and debate in the scientific literature for decades (Max, 1989; Randolph, 1956; Scott, 1983; Stall and Biernacki, 1986; Thorner, 1970). However, recent research using laboratory animal models suggests that overconsumption of certain food ingredients may engender addiction-like behaviors and neural adaptations, prompting a renewed interest in this topic. This chapter describes and explores research on the topic of food addiction, as well as discusses areas for future study.

DEFINING FEATURES

In the past decade, several researchers have explored the behavioral parallels between overeating and addiction to drugs of abuse. In 2007, Cassin and von Ranson conducted a seminal study on the subject, assessing addiction-like eating patterns among women with binge eating disorder (BED). The authors adapted the substance dependence criteria contained in the fourth edition of the *Diagnostic and Statistical Manual of Mental Disorders* (DSM-IV; American Psychiatric Association, 1994), replacing the term "substance" with "binge eating" (Goodman, 1990). Remarkably, 92.4% of participants met the DSM-IV substance dependence criteria, with the most frequently endorsed criteria being (1) binge eating larger amounts than intended, (2) continued binge eating despite knowledge of persistent adverse effects, and (3) a persistent desire or unsuccessful efforts to control binge eating (Cassin and von Ranson, 2007). These were the same criteria endorsed most often by individuals with BED in a recent qualitative study using the DSM-5 (American Psychiatric Association, 2013) substance use disorder (SUD) criteria, followed closely by the new criteria of craving (Curtis and Davis, 2014). Tolerance, in contrast, was one of the top three food-related SUD criteria endorsed by obese candidates for bariatric surgery (in addition to continued use despite the consequences and a persistent desire or repeated unsuccessful efforts to limit intake) (Meule et al., 2012a). Thus, although three or more of the seven DSM-IV-TR SUD criteria and evidence of clinically significant impairment are necessary to meet the criteria for a food addiction according to the Yale Food Addiction Scale (YFAS; discussed later), certain aspects of food addiction are more commonly reported and may thus be considered defining features of food addiction.

What distinguishes problematic overeating from overeating driven by addiction-like processes? When comparing overweight and obese women who reported compulsive overeating with or without food addiction, Bégin et al. (2012) observed three significant distinctions between the two groups: women with food addiction reported more severe binge eating, greater impulsivity, and less self-directedness (defined as the capacity to be effective, self-confident, and to act in accordance with personal goals). Notably, impulsivity scores did not differ significantly between those with food addiction and a third group of participants who had a SUD (and no food addiction). Koob and Volkow (2010) note that addiction includes both impulsivity and compulsivity; the former relates to behavior that is engaged in to experience feelings of pleasure (positive reinforcement), and the latter relates to behavior engaged in to avoid or attenuate stress or tension (negative reinforcement). This may explain why impulsivity was one of the key variables that differentiated women with a food addiction from other women seeking help for patterns of overeating that did not appear to involve an addictive component.

Neurobiology of Overeating and Food Addiction

Sugar and fat have both been shown independently to increase dopamine levels in brain regions associated with reward (Hajnal et al., 2004; Liang et al., 2006; Rada et al., 2012). In fact, whereas dopamine release typically wanes with repeated access to standard food, even palatable food such as sugar (Bassareo et al., 2015), it is elevated in response to sugar even after repeated exposure in sugar-bingeing animals, akin to the effect of drugs of abuse (Rada et al., 2005). The sugar-bingeing paradigm used in our laboratory (rats are food restricted for 12 hours/day and given access to both chow and sugar solutions for the remaining 12 hours) also leads to altered dopamine and opioid receptor binding (Colantuoni et al., 2001). With 3 weeks on this access schedule, rats demonstrate excessive consumption of the sugar solution during the first hour of access, constituting a "binge" episode (Avena et al., 2008). Following a history of bingeing, abstinence from sugar in sugar-preferring rats leads to increased effort to consume sugar when access is resumed (Avena et al., 2005), perhaps indicating craving or propensity to relapse. Rats maintained on the limited sugar access paradigm also show somatic signs of withdrawal, such as teeth chattering, head shakes, and forepaw tremors, following the administration of the opioid antagonist naloxone (Colantuoni et al., 2002).

Further evidence of behavioral and neural changes due to diet exposure comes from studies employing a cafeteria diet consisting of a variety of palatable food items, akin to our modern food environment. In one such study, rats fed a cafeteria diet exhibited dopamine release only in response to the cafeteria diet but not standard chow, unlike rats that were never exposed to this diet and exhibited dopamine release with chow alone (Geiger et al., 2009). Furthermore, exposure to a cafeteria diet is associated with weight gain and a downregulation of dopamine 2 (D2) receptors in rats (Johnson and Kenny, 2010). Decreased D2 receptors have been observed among individuals with obesity in some, but not all, studies, as well as among individuals with substance use disorders (see review by Murray et al., 2014).

Notably, cafeteria-fed rats also exhibit compulsive food intake behavior. Whereas control rats decrease their intake of palatable food in the presence of a cue indicating electric foot shock, rats with extended access to a cafeteria diet continue to consume the palatable food, suggesting that this behavior is impervious to the threat of adverse consequences (Johnson and Kenny, 2010). Similarly, rats identified as "binge-eating prone" will endure electric foot shocks at greater intensities than those considered "binge-eating resistant" in order to obtain palatable food (Oswald et al., 2011). Moreover, a recent study showed that rats were more resistant to the effects of punishment in the form of a mild foot shock when lever pressing for palatable food than for methamphetamine (Krasnova et al., 2014).

Neural correlates of food addiction have also been observed in humans when anticipating and receiving palatable food (Gearhardt et al., 2011a). Specifically, individuals with higher YFAS scores show heightened activation in brain areas associated with motivation to eat and craving anticipating the receipt of palatable food. However, these individuals exhibit less activation of the left lateral orbitofrontal cortex, a brain region associated with inhibition, during food consumption (Gearhardt et al., 2011a).

Research has also begun to investigate whether food addiction is associated with altered dopamine function in humans. In one such study, a composite score of multiple genetic markers indicated elevated dopamine signaling among those who met the YFAS criteria for food addiction compared to those who did not, providing preliminary evidence of a biological predisposition to problematic consumption of highly palatable foods due to a heightened reward response (Davis et al., 2013). Further evidence of perturbed dopamine functioning among those with food addiction comes from research showing that individuals with food addiction were resistant to the food-suppressing effect of a dopamine agonist relative to those who did not meet YFAS criteria for food addiction (Davis et al., 2014).

Collectively, these data indicate that in addition to eliciting behaviors that resemble addiction (e.g., bingeing and use despite adverse consequences), certain diets and intake patterns, particularly the overconsumption of highly palatable foods, can lead to neural responses in the short term (e.g., dopamine release) and neural adaptations over time (e.g., altered receptor binding) that may perpetuate unhealthy food intake habits and appear to parallel some of the neural effects seen with addiction to drugs of abuse.

METHODS FOR ASSESSMENT

The primary method available for assessing food addiction is a tool titled the Yale Food Addiction Scale. Developed by Ashley Gearhardt, William Corbin, and Kelly Brownell in 2009 at the Yale Rudd Center for Food Policy and Obesity, the YFAS is designed to identify individuals who exhibit signs of addictive behavior with regard to food (Gearhardt et al., 2009). The specific features of addiction measured by the YFAS are based on the substance dependence disorder criteria listed in the DSM-IV-TR (Box 8.1) as well as other assessment tools that have been used to study behavioral addictions, including the South Oaks Gambling Screen, the Exercise Dependence Scale, and the Carnes' Sexual Addiction Screening Tool (Gearhardt et al., 2009). The scale consists of 25 items (Table 8.1) answered using a Likert-type scale (i.e., never, once a month, 2–4 times a month, 2–3 times a week, or 4 or more times daily). Answers must meet designated thresholds to meet the criteria listed in Box 8.1. The YFAS has two scoring options—a symptom count and a dichotomous (yes/no) score. The latter requires that a participant has met three or more YFAS criteria and reports clinically significant impairment due to food/eating. The YFAS shows adequate internal reliability, good convergent validity, and fair discriminant validity (Gearhardt et al., 2009). Furthermore, French and Spanish versions of this scale show adequate to very good reliability, as well as good construct validity (Brunault et al., 2014; Granero et al., 2014). The YFAS has also been modified into an abbreviated version (mYFAS) (Flint et al., 2014) and a version for children (YFAS-C) (Gearhardt et al., 2013a).

PREVALENCE RATES

The prevalence of food addiction, according to studies using the YFAS, ranges from 4.0% in a sample of normal-weight female undergraduate students (Meule et al., 2012b) to 56.8% in a sample of adults with both obesity and BED (Gearhardt et al., 2012). Table 8.1 outlines prevalence rates across a variety of samples. In 2013, the first large-scale study using the YFAS was conducted in a sample of women participating in the Nurses Health Study II (NHS II). Among the 57,321 women included

Box 8.1

Sample Item for Each Criteria Included in the Yale Food Addiction Scale

Substance taken in larger amount and for longer period than intended
I find that when I start eating certain foods, I end up eating much more than planned.

Persistent desire or repeated unsuccessful attempts to quit
How many times in the past year did you try to cut down or stop eating certain foods altogether?

Much time/activity to obtain, use, recover
I spend a lot of time feeling sluggish or fatigued from overeating.

Important social, occupational, or recreational activities given up or reduced
There have been times when I consumed certain foods so often or in such large quantities that I started to eat food instead of working, spending time with my family or friends, or engaging in other important activities or recreational activities I enjoy.

Use continues despite knowledge of adverse consequences
I kept consuming the same types of food or the same amount of food even though I was having emotional and/or physical problems.

Tolerance
Over time, I have found that I need to eat more and more to get the feeling I want, such as reduced negative emotions or increased pleasure.

Withdrawal symptoms; substance taken to relieve withdrawal
I have had withdrawal symptoms such as agitation, anxiety, or other physical symptoms when I cut down or stopped eating certain foods. (Please do not include withdrawal symptoms caused by cutting down on caffeinated beverages such as soda pop, coffee, tea, energy drinks, etc.)

(continued)

Box 8.1 **Continued**

Use causes clinically significant impairment
I experience significant problems in my ability to function effectively (daily routine, job/school, social activities, family activities, health difficulties) because of food and eating.

in the analysis, 8.2% met the criteria for food addiction (Mason et al., 2013). In 2014, another study using the mYFAS in a sample of women in both the NHS and NHS II cohorts found that among the 134,175 women included in the analysis, 5.8% of participants met the criteria for food addiction (Flint et al., 2014). When divided by age, a greater percentage of the younger group in this study showed addictive-like relationships to food compared to the older group (8.4% vs. 2.7%, respectively). Given their size, these studies arguably provide the best estimates of the prevalence of food addiction among U.S. women. However, these samples differ from the general population with respect to several important characteristics, including gender and educational status; therefore, these rates may not accurately reflect rates in the general population, and relatively little is known about food addiction in nonclinical samples of men.

COMORBIDITIES

Studies with both large sample sizes and a wide range of body mass indexes (BMI) consistently report a positive relationship between food addiction and BMI, although smaller studies among samples with limited variation in BMI have not observed this association (Flint et al., 2014; Mason et al., 2013; Murphy et al., 2014; Pedram et al., 2013). Thus, in the general population, food addiction is most likely linked to higher body weight. In addition, and perhaps not surprisingly, there is considerable overlap between those who meet criteria for food addiction and those with eating disorder diagnoses, particularly BED and bulimia nervosa (BN) (Curtis and Davis, 2014; Davis et al., 2011; Gearhardt et al., 2012,

Table 8.1 PREVALENCE OF "FOOD ADDICTION" ACCORDING
TO THE YALE FOOD ADDICTION SCALE

Study	N	Sample Characteristics	% FA
Gearhardt et al. (2012)	81	Adults with obesity and BED	56.8
Clark and Saules (2013)[a]	67	Post-bariatric surgery patients	53.7[b]
Bégin et al. (2012)	23	Overweight and obese women seeking treatment	47.8
Meule et al. (2012a)	96	Obese bariatric surgery candidates	41.7
Gearhardt et al. (2013b)	96	Adults with obesity and BED	41.5
Meule et al. (2014a)	94	Obese weight loss surgery candidates	40.4
Gearhardt et al. (2011a)	39	Young healthy women	38.4[b]
Imperatori et al. (2014)	112	Overweight and obese adults seeking weight loss treatment	33.9
Pepino et al. (2014)	44	Obese adults seeking weight loss surgery	31.8
Davis et al. (2011)	72	Obese adults	25
Murphy et al. (2014)	233	Undergraduate students	24
Burmeister et al. (2013)	57	Overweight and obese adults	19.6[b]
Davis et al. (2013)	120	Men and women	17.5
Davis et al. (2014)	136	Predominately overweight and obese adults	16.9
Eichen et al. (2013)	178	Overweight and obese adults	15.2
Lent et al. (2014)	154	Adults seeking weight loss treatment	15.2
Gearhardt et al. (2009)	187–221	Undergraduate students	11.4
Meule et al. (2012c)	752	Young adults (predominately female students)	8.8
Brunault et al. (2014)	553	Nonclinical sample	8.7
Meule and Kubler (2012)	616	Young adults (predominately female students)	8.5
Mason et al. (2013)	57,321	Adult women	8.2
Gearhardt et al. (2013a)	72	Children and adolescents	7.2
Flint et al. (2014)	134,175	Adult women (Nurses' Health Studies I and II)	5.8
Pedram et al. (2013)	652	Adult men and women	5.4
Meule et al. (2012b)	50	Normal-weight female college students	4

[a]Retrospective data.
[b]Using the less stringent scoring option that requires three or more Yale Food Addiction Scale criteria but not clinically significant impairment.
BED, binge eating disorder; FA, meet criteria for food addiction.
Source: Adapted from Murray et al. (2014)

2013b, 2014; Meule et al., 2014b). In samples of those with BED, approximately half meet the criteria for food addiction as defined by the YFAS (Davis et al., 2011; Gearhardt et al., 2012), and these individuals tend to exhibit more severe pathology than those with BED alone (Gearhardt et al., 2012). Specifically, one study found that individuals with BED and food addiction report significantly more severe binge eating, depression, food cravings, and emotional, external, and hedonic eating, as well as greater impulsivity and more addictive personality traits, than those with BED but not food addiction (Davis, 2013). A qualitative study that adapted the most recent DSM-5 SUD criteria to food and eating found that all of the women with obesity and BED and approximately half of the women with obesity but not BED met the criteria for a food addiction (Curtis and Davis, 2014).

Like BED, BN is characterized in part by the presence of binge eating behavior, thus making it another population of interest in the study of food addiction. One study found that all of the women surveyed who had current BN met YFAS criteria for food addiction, in contrast to 30% of women in remission and 0% of controls (Meule et al., 2014b). Intriguingly, another study found higher rates of food addiction among those with BN than those with BED (Gearhardt et al., 2014). Furthermore, in another study, the percentage of individuals with BN who met Goodman's addictive disorder criteria was comparable to that found among individuals with substance disorders (Speranza et al., 2012). Research exploring possible differences in how "food addiction" is experienced by those with BN compared to those with BED may provide valuable insight into the construct of food addiction and how to best treat individuals with eating disorders who also report strong parallels between their eating and addiction. However, it is important to note that some have cautioned against comparing eating disorders too closely to an addictive disorder because this may distract from critical distinctions between these disorders (Cassin and von Ranson, 2007; Vandereycken, 1990). The identification of certain pathological behavioral patterns as addictive should serve to enhance our understanding and treatment of patients without taking away from the focus on other clinically relevant symptoms, which may not relate to addiction (e.g., body image disturbance). Thus, food addiction appears to be highly associated with eating disorders, and the question remains whether food addiction is a separate entity or a more severe subtype or variant of BED or BN. Nevertheless, studies have found participants without BED to meet the criteria for a food addiction (Davis et al., 2011), providing some evidence that addictive-like eating may be distinct from the currently recognized forms of pathological eating.

In terms of other psychiatric symptoms, food addiction has been associated with greater depressive symptomology (Burmeister et al., 2013; Davis et al., 2011; Eichen et al., 2013; Gearhardt et al., 2012; Meule et al., 2014a). Other psychological correlates of food addiction include increased negative affect, greater emotion dysregulation, and decreased self-esteem (Gearhardt et al., 2012, 2013b), as well as increased body shame (Burmeister et al., 2013). There are limited data regarding any potential comorbidity between food addiction and substance use disorders, and the extant data are mixed, with one study showing a positive correlation between problematic alcohol use and food addiction (Gearhardt et al., 2009) and another showing those with food addiction to report less evidence of alcohol use disorder (Meule, 2014a). Furthermore, another study found no relationship between problematic substance use and food addiction (Clark and Saules, 2013). Further research investigating the potential overlap between food addiction and other psychiatric disorders or symptoms may add to our current understanding of this construct.

RISK AND PROTECTIVE FACTORS

A systematic review identified three variables associated with food addiction: female gender, age (>35 years old), and overweight or obesity. Furthermore, as one might imagine, clinical samples tend to show higher rates of food addiction compared to nonclinical samples (Pursey et al.,

2014). It is worth noting that the potential role of socioeconomic status has not yet been explored with respect to food addiction.

As mentioned previously, a number of studies have observed a positive correlation between food addiction and impulsivity or facets of impulsivity (Bégin et al., 2012; Davis et al., 2011; Meule et al., 2012b, 2014a; Murphy et al., 2014), suggesting that this may be a potential risk factor for addictive-like eating. In addition, increased addictive traits, childhood attention deficit hyperactivity disorder, a younger age of first being overweight, and a younger age of dieting onset have all been related to food addiction (Davis et al., 2011; Gearhardt et al., 2013b). A history of severe physical and sexual abuse in childhood and adolescence has also been shown to increase the risk for food addiction in women in one study (Mason et al., 2013). Furthermore, higher food addiction rates have been reported among women with greater post-traumatic stress disorder (PTSD) symptoms (Mason et al., 2014).

Given the overlaps between impulsivity and addictive behavior (Grant and Chamberlain, 2014), as well as the frequency with which impulsivity has been observed among "food addicts," it is possible that this might also be a predisposing factor in the development of addictive-like eating. Notably, it has also been argued that engaging in addictive behavior may increase impulsivity, perhaps perpetuating this behavior (Grant and Chamberlain, 2014). In addition, increased emotion dysregulation, noted among those with higher food addiction scores (Gearhardt et al., 2013b), may lead to unhealthy ways of coping or responding to one's negative emotions (Bonn-Miller et al., 2008). Similarly, in light of the associations between food addiction and depression mentioned previously, and some research showing depressive symptomology to pre-date the onset of binge eating (Stice et al., 2002), depression is another potential risk factor for food addiction. It is conceivable that cycles of addictive-like eating may also lead to or exacerbate emotion dysregulation and depression. Thus, further research regarding the time course of such factors is needed to clarify psychological risk factors for food addiction.

TREATMENTS

Psychological Treatment

To date, no known empirical studies have been conducted to assess the efficacy of therapeutic interventions for overeating based on an addiction model. Interestingly, however, one survey found that approximately one-fourth of clinicians sampled employ an addiction-based therapy (including the 12-step approach) with eating disorder clients "often" or "always" (von Ranson and Robinson, 2006). When asked why, clinicians cited client preference, behavioral similarities between the two types of disorders, effectiveness based on clinical experience, and that this approach offered an additional means of support to clients. The potential benefit of this approach, however, remains unclear and warrants further research.

Insights regarding useful strategies for treating food addiction may be gleaned from existing therapeutic modalities used to treat BED, considering the significant overlap between the two noted previously. Cognitive behavioral therapy (CBT) is currently considered the preeminent treatment for BED and includes a number of features that may be helpful in the treatment of food addiction, including an emphasis on the adoption of healthy, alternative coping strategies as well as the identification of triggers. It has been proposed that a combination of techniques used in CBT for BED and CBT for substance dependence may be particularly well-suited for individuals with food addiction (Gearhardt et al., 2011b).

Although current treatments for BED may be helpful for those struggling with addictive-like eating, further research is needed to determine whether individuals identified as having a food addiction may respond well to, or perhaps show greater success with, other addiction-based treatment approaches. For example, Davis and Carter (2014) propose that treatment approaches that incorporate distress tolerance skill training, acceptance and mindfulness techniques with respect to food cravings, and cue exposure might be particularly beneficial for those struggling with addictive-like eating. Finally, in light of higher rates of food addiction among individuals who have experienced trauma and report PTSD symptoms, psychological interventions targeting addictive-like eating may benefit from considering the possible role of these factors in the development and maintenance of this behavioral pattern.

Pharmacological Treatment

Recent research has focused on exploring the efficacy of pharmacological agents known to target brain systems associated with reward (i.e., the dopaminergic and opioidergic systems) in suppressing overeating, particularly of highly palatable foods (Avena et al., 2013). Candidate pharmacological compounds include baclofen, a GABA-B agonist that has shown some promising results for the treatment of alcohol use disorder (Agabio and Colombo, 2014) and has been found to reduce binge eating in both preclinical and clinical studies (Berner et al., 2009; Broft et al., 2007; Buda-Levin et al., 2005; Corwin et al., 2012), as well as naltrexone, an opioid antagonist used to treat alcohol and opioid dependence (Modesto-Lowe and Van Kirk, 2002) and shown to reduce binge eating in several preclinical studies (Blasio et al., 2014; Corwin and Wojnicki, 2009; Giuliano et al., 2012; Rao et al., 2008; Wong et al., 2009). Recent preclinical work from our laboratory has found that 1 hour after administration, the combination of baclofen and naltrexone appears to be more effective in reducing intake of foods high in fat and fat/sugar combinations than either drug alone. Furthermore, the high dose of this combination did not significantly affect chow intake, indicating a selective suppression of intake of these palatable foods (Avena, Bocarsly, Murray, & Gold, 2014).

Given the overlaps between binge eating and addiction to drugs of abuse, our laboratory has also been interested in investigating the potential inhibitory effects of an aldehyde dehydrogenase 2 (ALDH2) inhibitor, shown to reduce self-administration of alcohol and cocaine in rats (Arolfo et al., 2009; Yao et al., 2010), on binge eating behavior. Results from our study in laboratory animals showed that the (ALDH2) inhibitor,

GS 455534, selectively reduced binge intake of sugar (vs. ad libitum intake of sugar), without affecting chow intake, as well as reduced binge intake of fat (vs. ad libitum intake of fat); however, in this case, chow intake was also decreased. Notably, GS 455534 also inhibited the normal dopamine release seen in the nucleus accumbens in response to sugar in sugar-bingeing rats, perhaps indicating the mechanism by which this compound works to suppress sugar overconsumption (Bocarsly et al., 2014).

Although neither psychological nor pharmacological, it is noteworthy to point out that remission of food addiction has been observed in the majority (93%) of previously identified "food-addicted" individuals following surgery-induced weight loss (Pepino et al., 2014). This is promising because studies show a high prevalence of food addiction among individuals seeking bariatric surgery (Clark and Saules, 2013; Meule et al., 2012a, 2014a). Like studies whether food addiction impacts weight loss in behavioral interventions (Burmeister et al., 2013; Lent et al., 2014), studies investigating the effect of food addiction on weight loss success following weight loss surgery have produced conflicting results (Clark and Saules, 2013; Pepino et al., 2014). Relatedly, there is evidence that food addiction "diagnoses" prior to surgery may be linked to greater problematic substance use post-surgery (Clark and Saules, 2013), a topic that warrants further attention.

Taken together, evidence in support of particular treatment strategies for food addiction is lacking. This is not surprising in light of the relative "infancy" of the empirical study of the food addiction construct. However, given the proliferation of studies assessing this construct in the past few years, research exploring the efficacy of different treatment modalities in this context seems a logical next step.

FUTURE DIRECTIONS

Although substantial work has been done to understand the behavioral characteristics and neural correlates of food addiction, many questions remain. Research directly comparing the effects of palatable food to drugs of abuse, for instance, would help to clarify the shared behavioral responses and brain adaptations as well as characterize possible distinctions. Moreover, additional research is needed to address existing gaps in the literature. For example, research is needed to determine whether food addiction is a separate disorder or a more severe form of other eating disorders. If it is determined to be a distinct condition, then greater research is needed to clarify the criteria for the condition and identify which criteria best align with, and which may not align well with, the criteria for substance use disorders. For instance, although there exist anecdotal reports of withdrawal symptoms when individuals abstain from particular types of foods or bingeing (Cassin and von Ranson, 2007; McAleavey and Fiumara, 2001), well-controlled studies are needed to determine whether predictable patterns of withdrawal emerge upon abstaining from palatable foods and whether this criterion is useful for the assessment of food addiction. Unique criteria related to the potential harm induced by excessive eating that may be distinct from those associated with substance use should be examined and may assist in classifying the condition. It is important to note that it is not necessary for food addiction to be entirely distinct from existing eating disorder diagnoses; rather, food addiction may accompany and be an underlying factor that contributes to and/or perpetuates pathological patterns of eating among those with eating disorder diagnoses. With this in mind, it may be relevant to investigate whether individuals who meet the criteria for a food addiction tend to report a longer duration of illness.

In light of the rates of food addiction seen in several clinical populations, it appears worthwhile to begin to explore whether psychological interventions specifically targeting addiction-like eating might confer benefits above and beyond current treatments of binge eating for individuals who identify as being "addicted" to food. Finally, an important next step is to explore the potential utility of prevention efforts at both the individual and societal levels, perhaps with interventions designed to help those who show greater risk for food addiction based on the literature discussed here.

REFERENCES

Agabio, R., Colombo, G., 2014. GABAB receptor ligands for the treatment of alcohol use disorder: Preclinical and clinical evidence. Front Neurosci. 8, 140.

American Psychiatric Association, 1994. Diagnostic and statistical manual of mental disorders (4th ed.). Washington, DC: American Psychiatric Association.

American Psychiatric Association, 2013. *Diagnostic and statistical manual of mental disorders* (5th ed.). Washington, DC: American Psychiatric Association.

Arolfo, M.P., Overstreet, D.H., Yao, L., Fan, P., Lawrence, A.J., Tao, G., et al., 2009. Suppression of heavy drinking and alcohol seeking by a selective ALDH-2 inhibitor. Alcohol Clin Exp Res. 33, 1935–1944.

Avena, N.M., Long, K.A., Hoebel, B.G., 2005. Sugar-dependent rats show enhanced responding for sugar after abstinence: Evidence of a sugar deprivation effect. Physiol Behav. 84, 359–362.

Avena, N.M., Rada, P., Hoebel, B.G., 2008. Evidence for sugar addiction: Behavioral and neurochemical effects of intermittent, excessive sugar intake. Neurosci Biobehav Rev. 32, 20–39.

Avena, N.M., Murray, S., Gold, M.S., 2013. The next generation of obesity treatments: Beyond suppressing appetite. Front Psychol. 4, 721.

Avena, N.M., Bocarsly, M.E., Murray, S., Gold, M.S., 2014. Effects of baclofen and naltrexone, alone and in combination, on the consumption of palatable food in male rats. Exp Clin Psychopharmacol. 22(5):460–467. doi: 10.1037/a0037223. Epub 2014 Jul 28.

Bassareo, V., Cucca, F., Musio, P., Lecca, D., Frau, R., Di Chiara, G. 2015. Nucleus accumbens shell and core dopamine responsiveness to sucrose in rats: role of response contingency and discriminative/conditioned cues. The European Journal of Neuroscience.

Bégin, C., St-Louis, M., Turmel, S., Tousignant, B., Marion, L., Ferland, F., et al., 2012. Does food addiction distinguish a specific subgroup of overweight/obese overeating women? Health. 4, 1492–1499.

Berner, L.A., Bocarsly, M.E., Hoebel, B.G., Avena, N.M., 2009. Baclofen suppresses binge eating of pure fat but not a sugar-rich or sweet-fat diet. Behav Pharmacol. 20, 631–634.

Blasio, A., Steardo, L., Sabino, V., Cottone, P., 2014. Opioid system in the medial prefrontal cortex mediates binge-like eating. Addict Biol. 19, 652–662.

Bocarsly, M.E., Hoebel, B.G., Paredes, D., von Loga, I., Murray, S.M., Wang, M., et al., 2014. GS 455534 selectively suppresses binge eating of palatable food and attenuates dopamine release in the accumbens of sugar-bingeing rats. Behav Pharmacol. 25, 147–157.

Bonn-Miller, M.O., Vujanovic, A.A., Zvolensky, M.J., 2008. Emotional dysregulation: Association with coping-oriented marijuana use motives among current marijuana users. Subst Use Misuse. 43, 1653–1665.

Broft, A.I., Spanos, A., Corwin, R.L., Mayer, L., Steinglass, J., Devlin, M.J., et al., 2007. Baclofen for binge eating: An open-label trial. Int J Eat Disord. 40, 687–691.

Brunault, P., Ballon, N., Gaillard, P., Reveillere, C., Courtois, R., 2014. Validation of the French version of the Yale Food Addiction Scale: An examination of its factor structure, reliability, and construct validity in a nonclinical sample. Can J Psychiatry. 59, 276–284.

Buda-Levin, A., Wojnicki, F.H., Corwin, R.L., 2005. Baclofen reduces fat intake under binge-type conditions. Physiol Behav. 86, 176–184.

Burmeister, J.M., Hinman, N., Koball, A., Hoffmann, D.A., Carels, R.A., 2013. Food addiction in adults seeking weight loss treatment: Implications for psychosocial health and weight loss. Appetite. 60, 103–110.

Cassin, S.E., von Ranson, K.M., 2007. Is binge eating experienced as an addiction? Appetite. 49, 687–690.

Clark, S.M., Saules, K.K., 2013. Validation of the Yale Food Addiction Scale among a weight-loss surgery population. Eat Behav. 14, 216–219.

Colantuoni, C., Schwenker, J., McCarthy, J., Rada, P., Ladenheim, B., Cadet, J.L., et al., 2001. Excessive sugar intake alters binding to dopamine and mu-opioid receptors in the brain. Neuroreport. 12, 3549–3552.

Colantuoni, C., Rada, P., McCarthy, J., Patten, C., Avena, N.M., Chadeayne, A., et al., 2002. Evidence that intermittent, excessive sugar intake causes endogenous opioid dependence. Obes Res. 10, 478–88.

Corwin, R.L., Wojnicki, F.H., 2009. Baclofen, raclopride, and naltrexone differentially affect intake of fat and sucrose under limited access conditions. Behav Pharmacol. 20, 537–548.

Corwin, R.L., Boan, J., Peters, K.F., Ulbrecht, J.S., 2012. Baclofen reduces binge eating in a double-blind, placebo-controlled, crossover study. Behav Pharmacol. 23, 616–625.

Curtis, C., Davis, C., 2014. A qualitative study of binge eating and obesity from an addiction perspective. Eat Disord. 22, 19–32.

Davis, C., 2013. Compulsive overeating as an addictive behavior: Overlap between food addiction and binge eating disorder. Curr Obes Rep. 2, 171–178.

Davis, C., Carter, J.C., 2014. If certain foods are addictive, how might this change the treatment of compulsive overeating and obesity? Curr Addict Rep. 1, 89–95.

Davis, C., Curtis, C., Levitan, R.D., Carter, J.C., Kaplan, A.S., Kennedy, J.L., 2011. Evidence that "food addiction" is a valid phenotype of obesity. Appetite. 57, 711–717.

Davis, C., Loxton, N.J., Levitan, R.D., Kaplan, A.S., Carter, J.C., Kennedy, J.L., 2013. "Food addiction" and its association with a dopaminergic multilocus genetic profile. Physiol Behav. 118, 63–69.

Davis, C., Levitan, R.D., Kaplan, A.S., Kennedy, J.L., Carter, J.C., 2014. Food cravings, appetite, and snack-food consumption in response to a psychomotor stimulant drug: The moderating effect of "food-addiction." Front Psychol. 5, 403.

Eichen, D.M., Lent, M.R., Goldbacher, E., Foster, G.D., 2013. Exploration of "food addiction" in overweight and obese treatment-seeking adults. Appetite. 67, 22–24.

Flint, A.J., Gearhardt, A.N., Corbin, W.R., Brownell, K.D., Field, A.E., Rimm, E.B., 2014. Food-addiction scale measurement in 2 cohorts of middle-aged and older women. Am J Clin Nutr. 99, 578–586.

Gearhardt, A.N., Corbin, W.R., Brownell, K.D., 2009. Preliminary validation of the Yale Food Addiction Scale. Appetite. 52, 430–436.

Gearhardt, A.N., Yokum, S., Orr, P.T., Stice, E., Corbin, W.R., Brownell, K.D., 2011a. Neural correlates of food addiction. Arch Gen Psychiatry. 68, 808–816.

Gearhardt, A.N., White, M.A., Potenza, M.N., 2011b. Binge eating disorder and food addiction. Curr Drug Abuse Rev. 4, 201–207.

Gearhardt, A.N., White, M.A., Masheb, R.M., Morgan, P.T., Crosby, R.D., Grilo, C.M., 2012. An examination of the food addiction construct in obese patients with binge eating disorder. Int J Eat Disord. 45, 657–663.

Gearhardt, A.N., Roberto, C.A., Seamans, M.J., Corbin, W.R., Brownell, K.D., 2013a. Preliminary validation of the Yale Food Addiction Scale for children. Eat Behav. 14, 508–512.

Gearhardt, A.N., White, M.A., Masheb, R.M., Grilo, C.M., 2013b. An examination of food addiction in a racially diverse sample of obese patients with binge eating disorder in primary care settings. Compr Psychiatry. 54, 500–505.

Gearhardt, A.N., Boswell, R.G., White, M.A., 2014. The association of "food addiction" with disordered eating and body mass index. Eat Behav. 15, 427–433.

Geiger, B.M., Haburcak, M., Avena, N.M., Moyer, M.C., Hoebel, B.G., Pothos, E.N., 2009. Deficits of mesolimbic dopamine neurotransmission in rat dietary obesity. Neuroscience. 159, 1193–1199.

Giuliano, C., Robbins, T.W., Nathan, P.J., Bullmore, E.T., Everitt, B.J., 2012. Inhibition of opioid transmission at the mu-opioid receptor prevents both food seeking and binge-like eating. Neuropsychopharmacology. 37, 2643–2652.

Goodman, A., 1990. Addiction: Definition and implications. Br J Addict. 85, 1403–1408.

Granero, R., Hilker, I., Aguera, Z., Jimenez-Murcia, S., Sauchelli, S., Islam, M.A., et al., 2014. Food addiction in a Spanish sample of eating disorders: DSM-5 diagnostic subtype differentiation and validation data. Eur Eat Disord Rev. 22, 389–396.

Grant, J.E., Chamberlain, S.R., 2014. Impulsive action and impulsive choice across substance and behavioral addictions: Cause or consequence? Addict Behav. 39, 1632–1639.

Hajnal, A., Smith, G.P., Norgren, R., 2004. Oral sucrose stimulation increases accumbens dopamine in the rat. Am J Physiol Regul Integr Comp Physiol. 286, R31–R37.

Ifland, J.R., Preuss, H.G., Marcus, M.T., Rourke, K.M., Taylor, W.C., Burau, K., et al., 2009. Refined food addiction: A classic substance use disorder. Med Hypotheses. 72, 518–526.

Imperatori, C., Innamorati, M., Contardi, A., Continisio, M., Tamburello, S., Lamis, D.A., et al., 2014. The association among food addiction, binge eating severity and psychopathology in obese and overweight patients attending low-energy-diet therapy. Compr Psychiatry. 55, 1358–1362.

Johnson, P.M., Kenny, P.J., 2010. Dopamine D2 receptors in addiction-like reward dysfunction and compulsive eating in obese rats. Nat Neurosci. 13, 635–641.

Koob, G.F., Volkow, N.D., 2010. Neurocircuitry of addiction. Neuropsychopharmacology. 35, 217–238.

Krasnova, I.N., Marchant, N.J., Ladenheim, B., McCoy, M.T., Panlilio, L.V., Bossert, J.M., et al., 2014. Incubation of methamphetamine and palatable food craving after punishment-induced abstinence. Neuropsychopharmacology. 39, 2008–2016.

Lent, M.R., Eichen, D.M., Goldbacher, E., Wadden, T.A., Foster, G.D., 2014. Relationship of food addiction to weight loss and attrition during obesity treatment. Obesity (Silver Spring). 22, 52–55.

Liang, N.C., Hajnal, A., Norgren, R., 2006. Sham feeding corn oil increases accumbens dopamine in the rat. Am J Physiol Regul Integr Comp Physiol. 291, R1236–R1239.

Mason, S.M., Flint, A.J., Field, A.E., Austin, S.B., Rich-Edwards, J.W., 2013. Abuse victimization in childhood or adolescence and risk of food addiction in adult women. Obesity (Silver Spring). 21, E775–E781.

Mason, S.M., Flint, A.J., Roberts, A.L., Agnew-Blais, J., Koenen, K.C., Rich-Edwards, J.W., 2014. Posttraumatic stress disorder symptoms and food addiction in women by timing and type of trauma exposure. JAMA Psychiatry. 71, 1271–1278.

Max, B., 1989. This and that: Chocolate addiction, the dual pharmacogenetics of asparagus eaters, and the arithmetic of freedom. Trends Pharmacol Sci. 10, 390–393.

McAleavey, K.M.A., Fiumara, M.C., 2001. Eating disorders: Are they addictions? A dialogue. J Soc Work Pract Addict. 1, 107–113.

Meule, A., Kubler, A., 2012. Food cravings in food addiction: The distinct role of positive reinforcement. Eat Behav. 13, 252–255.

Meule, A., Heckel, D., Kubler, A., 2012a. Factor structure and item analysis of the Yale Food Addiction Scale in obese candidates for bariatric surgery. Eur Eat Disord Rev. 20, 419–422.

Meule, A., Lutz, A., Vogele, C., Kubler, A., 2012b. Women with elevated food addiction symptoms show accelerated reactions, but no impaired inhibitory control, in response to pictures of high-calorie food-cues. Eat Behav. 13, 423–428.

Meule, A., Vogele, C., Kubler, A., 2012c. [German translation and validation of the Yale Food Addiction Scale]. Diagnostica. 58, 115–126.

Meule, A., Heckel, D., Jurowich, C., Vogele, C., Kubler, A., 2014a. Correlates of food addiction in obese individuals seeking bariatric surgery. Clin Obesity. 4, 228–236.

Meule, A., von Rezori, V., Blechert, J., 2014b. Food addiction and bulimia nervosa. Eur Eat Disord Rev. 22, 331–337.

Modesto-Lowe, V., Van Kirk, J., 2002. Clinical uses of naltrexone: A review of the evidence. Exp Clin Psychopharmacol. 10, 213–227.

Murphy, C.M., Stojek, M.K., MacKillop, J., 2014. Interrelationships among impulsive personality traits, food addiction, and body mass index. Appetite. 73, 45–50.

Murray, S., Tulloch, A., Gold, M.S., Avena, N.M., 2014. Hormonal and neural mechanisms of food reward, eating behaviour and obesity. Nat Rev Endocrinol. 10, 540–552.

Oswald, K.D., Murdaugh, D.L., King, V.L., Boggiano, M.M., 2011. Motivation for palatable food despite consequences in an animal model of binge eating. Int J Eat Disord. 44, 203–211.

Pedram, P., Wadden, D., Amini, P., Gulliver, W., Randell, E., Cahill, F., et al., 2013. Food addiction: Its prevalence and significant association with obesity in the general population. PLoS One. 8, e74832.

Pepino, M.Y., Stein, R.I., Eagon, J.C., Klein, S., 2014. Bariatric surgery-induced weight loss causes remission of food addiction in extreme obesity. Obesity (Silver Spring). 22, 1792–1798.

Pursey, K.M., Stanwell, P., Gearhardt, A.N., Collins, C.E., Burrows, T.L., 2014. The prevalence of food addiction as assessed by the Yale Food Addiction Scale: A systematic review. Nutrients. 6, 4552–4590.

Rada, P., Avena, N.M., Hoebel, B.G., 2005. Daily bingeing on sugar repeatedly releases dopamine in the accumbens shell. Neuroscience. 134, 737–744.

Rada, P., Avena, N.M., Barson, J.R., Hoebel, B.G., Leibowitz, S.F., 2012. A high-fat meal, or intraperitoneal administration of a fat emulsion, increases extracellular dopamine in the nucleus accumbens. Brain Sci. 2, 242–253.

Randolph, T.G., 1956. The descriptive features of food addiction; Addictive eating and drinking. Q J Stud Alcohol. 17, 198–224.

Rao, R.E., Wojnicki, F.H., Coupland, J., Ghosh, S., Corwin, R.L., 2008. Baclofen, raclopride, and naltrexone differentially reduce solid fat emulsion intake under limited access conditions. Pharmacol Biochem Behav. 89, 581–590.

Scott, D.W., 1983. Alcohol and food abuse: Some comparisons. Br J Addict. 78, 339–349.

Speranza, M., Revah-Levy, A., Giquel, L., Loas, G., Venisse, J.L., Jeammet, P., et al., 2012. An investigation of Goodman's addictive disorder criteria in eating disorders. Eur Eat Disord Rev. 20, 182–189.

Stall, R., Biernacki, P., 1986. Spontaneous remission from the problematic use of substances: An inductive model derived from a comparative analysis of the alcohol, opiate, tobacco, and food/obesity literatures. Int J Addict. 21, 1–23.

Stice, E., Presnell, K., Spangler, D., 2002. Risk factors for binge eating onset in adolescent girls: A 2-year prospective investigation. Health Psychol. 21, 131–138.

Thorner, H.A., 1970. On compulsive eating. J Psychosom Res. 14, 321–325.

Vandereycken, W., 1990. The addiction model in eating disorders: Some critical remarks and a selected bibliography. Int J Eat Disord. 9, 95–101.

von Ranson, K.M., Robinson, K.E., 2006. Who is providing what type of psychotherapy to eating disorder clients? A survey. Int J Eat Disord. 39, 27–34.

Wong, K.J., Wojnicki, F.H., Corwin, R.L., 2009. Baclofen, raclopride, and naltrexone differentially affect intake of fat/sucrose mixtures under limited access conditions. Pharmacol Biochem Behav. 92, 528–536.

Yao, L., Fan, P., Arolfo, M., Jiang, Z., Olive, M.F., Zablocki, J., et al., 2010. Inhibition of aldehyde dehydrogenase-2 suppresses cocaine seeking by generating THP, a cocaine use-dependent inhibitor of dopamine synthesis. Nat Med. 16, 1024–1028.

9

Addicted to UV

Evidence for Tanning Addiction

JEROD L. STAPLETON, JOEL HILLHOUSE,
AND ELLIOT J. COUPS ∎

In 2012, Patricia Krentcil made headlines as the "Tanning Mom" accused of endangering her 6-year-old daughter by illegally allowing the girl to use an ultraviolet radiation (UVR)-emitting tanning bed. Although Ms. Krentcil was never criminally charged for the alleged incident, she appeared in several highly visible media outlets and became well-known for her shocking burnt-orange skin and professed lifelong love of tanning (Chan, 2012; Davis and Riley, 2012). The term "tanoxeria" became popular in the media to describe such behavior that seemed to reflect an addiction to tanning. This chapter reviews scientific studies of tanning behavior to determine the empirical evidence regarding the potential addictive qualities of tanning.

Tanning is defined as intentional, intermittent UVR exposure in the form of lying in the sun (i.e., sunbathing) or through the use of indoor tanning beds and lamps that emit artificial UVR (i.e., indoor tanning). Occasional tanning is a common behavior for individuals seeking the cosmetic effects of tanning, in the form of increased skin pigmentation and a darker skin appearance. However, the excessive tanning behavior of some individuals seems to exceed the amount of exposure necessary to maintain a tanned appearance. For example, Poorsattar and Hornung (2007) found that 9% of participants in a college undergraduate sample tanned outdoors or indoors 20 times or more in the previous month. Some have speculated that these frequent tanners may be experiencing addictive-like symptoms of tanning, and a small body of empirical studies of tanning addiction has emerged during the past decade.

Changes in the fifth edition of the *Diagnostic and Statistical Manual of Mental Disorders* (DSM-5; American Psychiatric Association, 2013) resulted in broadening the definition of addiction to "Substance-Related and Addictive Disorders." This change opens the possibility for the recognition of non-substance behavioral addictions (American Psychiatric Association, 2013), although empirical evidence of defining characteristics that relate to clinically significant harms is needed prior to recognition of any condition as a psychiatric disorder. The small body of tanning addiction research does not yet present the type of compelling body of empirical evidence that would lead to an official recognition of tanning addiction as a psychiatric condition. This is not unexpected given that tanning addiction research is in its formative stage and has been conducted only during approximately the past decade. Indeed, research on gambling disorder has existed for decades, and it had previously been included in earlier versions of the DSM as an impulse control disorder. Research conducted during the past 15 years set the stage to align gambling disorder alongside substance use disorders as the first non-substance use addiction. The current literature on tanning appears to provide preliminary support for expanding research efforts into tanning addiction as a mental disorder in general and as a behavioral addiction in particular. The strongest evidence for tanning addiction comes from lab, mouse, and human experimental studies that suggest the physiological effect of UVR exposure during tanning can activate biological reward pathways in ways that are similar to those observed in substance use disorders. This chapter reviews the evidence for tanning addiction and proposes future research directions that could help to bolster the evidence regarding tanning addiction and fill in critical evidence gaps.

DEFINING FEATURES

To better evaluate the body of evidence for tanning addiction, we first define a behavioral addiction framework that reflects the DSM-5 and the conceptual model presented by Grant and colleagues (2010). The case for considering tanning as a behavioral addiction would be strengthened by demonstrating shared similarities with these models of addiction. Within this framework, addiction represents increasingly impaired control over the use of a substance or a behavior that becomes problematic to an individual over time. For an individual with a substance use disorder, the behavior initially provides short-term, pleasurable feelings. These pleasurable feelings are a result of the activation of dopaminergic reward pathways and endorphin release. Feelings of euphoria and increased mood with activation of these pathways are behaviorally reinforced and conditioned with each use of the drug. Therefore, a compelling physiological basis for tanning addiction would include evidence for a biological reward pathway with tanning. Over time, repeated behavior engagement and stimulation of reward pathways may lead to physiological changes that reduce the pleasure associated with the behavior. This reduction in pleasure is termed tolerance, and it results in more frequent or prolonged behavior in an attempt to re-create the rewarding feelings. In the case of physiological dependence, the behavior becomes motivated by the need for relief from symptoms of withdrawal. Tolerance and withdrawal are hallmarks of substance use disorders.

Physical dependence is a critical process in the development of some substance use disorders. However, physiological dependence on a substance does not imply addiction unless it is accompanied by behaviors that are disruptive, harmful, or cause problems for an individual. The defining aspects of behavioral addiction are lack of control over the behavior to the point of becoming problematic (American Psychiatric Association, 2013; Grant et al., 2010). Thus, behavioral addictions are manifest in significant psychological, social, and health problems from repetitive engagement in the behavior. A strong case for tanning as an addiction requires evidence that the experience of tanning addiction is similar to the experience of other addictions in these critical ways.

There is a need for a conceptualization of the defining features and symptoms of tanning addiction based on this behavioral addiction framework:

Proposed Defining Features and Symptoms of Tanning Addiction

1. Often tans when feeling distressed or in a bad mood
2. Experiences desires, urges, or cravings to go tanning
3. Has increased frequency of tanning in order to get desired affective benefits of tanning
4. Is restless or irritable when attempting to cut down or stop tanning
5. Has made repeated unsuccessful attempts to control, reduce, or stop tanning
6. Is often preoccupied with thinking about tanning
7. Has given up or not met important social, educational, or career activities/obligations because of time or other resources spent on tanning
8. Continues tanning despite recurrent psychological or physical problems with tanning (e.g., sunburns, skin cancer, or recurrent concerns about safety or health)

Preliminary evidence for each of these features can be found in the various studies of tanning addiction described throughout this chapter. There remains a need for phenomenological studies to identify the clinical characteristics of tanning addiction as described by tanners in order to fully evaluate this conceptualization of tanning addiction.

A PHYSIOLOGICAL MECHANISM FOR TANNING ADDICTION: ENDOGENOUS ENDORPHINS

It is important to present evidence of the biological effects of possible behavioral addictions in order to establish the potential for the behavior to transition from a rewarding, pleasurable experience to one that results in symptoms of physical dependence and the resulting significant personal problems and distress. The most compelling evidence of the addictive potential of tanning comes from in vitro studies of a possible mechanism for a biological UVR reward pathway. UVR can induce an endorphin response that is similar to the response to some substances of abuse. The biological mechanism for tanning addiction is most likely the release of endogenous opioids as a by-product of the skin response to UVR (Cui et al., 2007; Fell et al., 2014; Gilchrest et al., 1996; Schauer et al., 1994; Wintzen et al., 2001). UVR irradiation causes skin cell DNA damage. This damage induces a skin pigmentation process that begins with activation of the tumor suppressor protein p53 and the induction of pro-opiomelanocortin (POMC) production in skin keratinocytes (Cui et al., 2007; Wintzen et al., 2001). The derivatives of POMC include β-endorphin, an endogenous opioid, and adrenocorticotrophic hormone (ACTH). The demonstration that POMC is produced directly from the skin following UVR exposure is a novel finding because it was previously thought that the protein and its derivatives were produced primarily in the pituitary gland (Shah et al., 2012). These β-endorphins act locally on the skin by alleviating the skin irritation and inflammation associated with UVR overexposure (Cui et al., 2007). β-Endorphin is also an agonist to receptors that receive the active chemicals produced with ingestion of opium-derived drugs, and it has been shown to induce analgesia and euphoria (Roth-Deri et al., 2008). To the extent that β-endorphins produced by UVR exposure act on the central nervous system, it is possible that these hormones could contribute to the development of tanning addiction. Efforts to demonstrate that UVR exposure results in increased serum levels of endorphins with in vivo human studies, however, have provided inconsistent results (Gambichler et al., 2002; Kaur et al., 2005; Levins et al., 1983; Wintzen et al., 2001), providing only modest support for an endogenous opioid hypothesis of tanning addiction.

Evidence for a Tanning Reward Pathway

Feldman and colleagues (2004) conducted an experimental study of the rewarding properties of tanning. The researchers recruited 14 regular indoor tanning bed users and assigned each to alternately use one of two commercially available tanning beds. The tanning beds were identical with the exception that one was a sham bed with a filter that blocked UVR. Given that the beds appeared identical and both provided a warm, quiet tanning experience, any preference observed for the UVR bed over the UVR-sham bed was hypothesized to be due to the activation of biological reward pathways from UVR exposure.

Feldman et al.'s (2004) study followed a weekly protocol during a 6-week period. On Mondays and Wednesdays, the participants used both beds in a randomly assigned order and completed mood ratings following use of each bed. Participants reported greater relaxation and lower perceived tension following the use of the UVR bed compared to the sham bed. They also liked the UVR bed better overall. No differences were reported in other mood states, including feeling sad, distressed, enthusiastic, irritable, or nervous. On Fridays, participants were allowed to choose whether they wanted to tan and, if they did tan, which bed they would use. Participants chose the bed that emitted UVR over the sham bed on 95% of these occasions. The preference for the UVR in this study provides indirect evidence of the physiological effect of tanning through a biological reward pathway.

Harrington and colleagues (2012) explored the reinforcing properties of UVR in their study of UVR exposure-induced brain activity. They utilized Feldman et al.'s (2004) experimental approach of exposing participants to both a UVR and a sham tanning bed. Eligible participants had used a tanning bed at least two times per week for the past 90 days and scored positively on a screening assessment of tanning addiction symptoms. Participants' regional cerebral blood flow was assessed with single-photon emission computed technology (SPECT) during use of each tanning bed. Blood flow increases were observed in areas of the brain associated with drug-induced reward during the UVR bed session. Specifically, UVR tanning sessions resulted in increases in regional cerebral blood flow of the dorsal striatum, anterior insula, and medial orbitofunctional cortex relative to the sham session. Participants were significantly more likely to report a reduced desire to tan following a session in the UVR bed compared to the UVR-filtered bed. This finding is consistent with the earlier work of Feldman and colleagues (2004). This study provided the first evidence that UVR exposure can activate central neural dopamine pathways.

An experimental study by Kaur and colleagues (2006) expanded Feldman et al.'s (2004) work by indirectly demonstrating a role of endogenous opioids in the experience of tanning reward. Frequent tanners may be expected to have chronically elevated levels of opioids from tanning and upregulation of opioid receptors. Kaur and colleagues tested whether the administration of naltrexone, a narcotic antagonist that binds to central and peripheral opioid receptors, would block the preference for UVR tanning beds observed in Feldman and colleagues' (2004) experiment. Participants were exposed to tanning sessions in both UVR tanning beds and sham beds. Participants were 16 users of indoor tanning beds divided into two groups of either frequent tanners (defined as using indoor tanning 8–15 times a month) or infrequent tanners (defined as using indoor tanning in the past but not more than 12 times in any given year). Exposure condition was blinded to participants, and the order of exposure was varied randomly. Prior to exposure, participants were randomly assigned to receive a dose of naltrexone (5, 15, or 25 mg) or placebo. Following exposure, participants were asked to indicate their tanning bed preference. When placebo was administered, frequent tanners had a stronger preference for the UVR bed over the sham bed compared to infrequent tanners. The greater sensitivity to the effects of UVR among frequent tanners could reflect an upregulation of opioid receptors from chronic exposure to endogenous opioids. This finding held at the lowest level of naltrexone administration. However, the preference for the UVR bed among frequent tanners was greatly reduced at the two highest levels of naltrexone administration. The reduction of positive effects of tanning with blockage of opioid binding sites provided the first indirect evidence of an endogenous opioid pathway in the reinforcing effects of tanning. Perhaps even more telling was that 4 of 8 frequent tanner participants observed adverse effects (i.e., nausea and/or jitteriness) upon administration of the mid-level dose of naltrexone. Two of these participants withdrew early from the study because of these effects. No adverse effects were reported by infrequent tanners. The same research group found similar adverse effects of naltrexone among frequent tanners in a previous pilot study (Kaur et al., 2005). The withdrawal-like symptoms observed among the frequent tanners are similar to, but less severe than, symptoms observed when the drug is administered to individuals with physiological dependence on opioids, suggesting that frequent tanners may have chronically elevated levels of endogenous opioids.

A Mouse Model of Tanning Addiction

Fell and colleagues (2014) developed a novel mouse model of tanning addiction that supports and expands the human experimental studies. This group exposed mice to levels of UVR for 6 weeks that would be comparable to a human spending 20 to 30 minutes in the midday sun in Florida 5 days per week. Plasma endorphin levels were elevated within 1 week among the UVR-exposed mice compared to control mice, and they remained elevated during the 6-week study. These increases have been difficult to demonstrate in human studies of UVR exposure. UVR-exposed mice exhibited a rigidity of the tail that is typically seen in mice conditioned to be addicted to substances. There was also evidence that UVR-exposed mice had higher thresholds to mechanical- and thermal-induced pain, and these thresholds were reduced upon administration of naloxone, a short-acting version of naltrexone. β-Endorphin knockout mice displayed no changes in such thresholds. The authors also found evidence of the role of induction of p53-mediated POMC production by skin keratinocytes in the development of tanning addiction. Mice lacking p53 POMC production did not exhibit a skin tanning response and did not have increases in endorphins or pain thresholds following the UVR exposure schedule.

This study also provided preliminary evidence of the potential for tolerance to UVR. Tolerance was assessed by the evaluation of cross-tolerance with morphine. Mice were exposed to a hot plate and provided access to morphine, which could be self-administered to provide analgesic effects. UVR-exposed mice self-administered significantly higher levels of morphine during the hot plate exposure compared to control mice. The UVR mice may have developed opioid tolerance from the UVR exposure and required more morphine to reduce the pain of the hot plate test. Fell et al. (2014) also demonstrated evidence of dependence to UVR. UVR-exposed mice displayed classic symptoms of opioid withdrawal when administered naloxone. These symptoms were considered by the authors to be smaller in magnitude than symptoms typically observed with substances. UVR-exposed mice were also conditioned to avoid environments in which naloxone was administered, likely due to the withdrawal experienced within such environments. These findings both support and expand an opioid model of tanning addiction.

Summary of the Physiological Evidence of Tanning Addiction

Taken as a whole, the physiological literature provides compelling but preliminary evidence that UVR exposure during tanning can be biologically reinforcing. In vitro studies provide evidence that a likely mechanism for tanning dependence is the UVR exposure-induced production of endogenous opioids. A mouse model study of tanning addiction provides a variety of evidence that supports this view. Tanners in experimental clinical studies report stronger rewarding effects of UVR-emitting tanning beds compared to sham beds. Frequent tanners may react poorly to the administration of an opioid blocking drug, a response observed in individuals with opioid dependence. This suggests that frequent tanners may have chronically elevated levels of endogenous opioids, presumably as a result of excessive tanning.

Although intriguing, it is important to note the limitations of these studies. First, the evidence is based on a small number of studies, and the generalizability of the findings remains to be determined. These studies need to be replicated and expanded in additional samples with more diverse tanning experiences. Only one brain imaging study has been published, resulting in a limited understanding of how UVR exposure influences physiological responses. Future imaging studies should be conducted to determine how excessive tanning can lead to physiological changes in the brain or in the expression of opioid receptors.

THE EXPERIENCE OF TANNING ADDICTION

If tanning is an addiction, it is important to demonstrate that the experience of excessive tanning mirrors that of other addictions in terms of engendering an inability to control tanning behavior and physical or psychological problems. There is preliminary evidence of some similarities between the experience of tanning addiction and other substance use and behavioral addictions. Hillhouse and colleagues (2012) developed an assessment for tanning addiction, called the Structured Interview of Tanning Abuse and Dependence (SITAD), based on the Structured Clinical Interview for DSM-IV Axis 1 disorders for opiate use disorder. The SITAD was administered to a sample of 296 undergraduate students. Approximately 5% of the sample met three or more criteria, such as a loss of control over tanning, a desire to cut down, preoccupation or psychological problems with tanning, or symptoms of tolerance or withdrawal from tanning. These participants reported nearly 10 times more tanning sessions during a 6-month period compared to participants who did not meet these criteria. An additional 11% of the sample experienced some personal or social problems related to tanning but not multiple symptoms. A complete description of the SITAD is presented later.

The experience of behavioral addiction includes an inability to control behavior, which causes physical or psychological problems or harm to the individual or others. Survey research provides some limited information regarding the experience of tanning addiction. Lack of control in behavioral addictions can be evidenced by a difficulty in resisting a behavior or with unsuccessful attempts to reduce a behavior (Grant et al., 2010). Zeller and colleagues (2006) surveyed past year indoor tanning users aged 14 to 17 years regarding how difficult it would be for them to stop using indoor tanning. Nearly 1 in 3 individuals reported that they would find it difficult to quit tanning. Participants who used tanning frequently and started tanning at a younger age were more likely to report perceived difficulty in quitting tanning. Harrington and colleagues (2011) surveyed tanners who used indoor tanning at least three times per week and found that 21% believed they should stop or decrease their tanning and 9% had tried to stop tanning but were unsuccessful. In another study, 10% of undergraduate student tanners wanted to stop tanning but believed that they could not (Ashrafioun and Bonar, 2014b). Several studies present evidence that between 10% and 33% of tanners report feeling guilty that they tan too much (Harrington et al., 2011; Mosher and Danoff-Burg, 2010; Poorsattar and Hornung, 2007). The experience of guilt related to overuse of tanning suggests that these tanners view their use of tanning as personally unacceptable.

Although some frequent tanners experience guilt related to their tanning and may wish to reduce it, there are very few studies that clearly document psychological and interpersonal problems associated with tanning addiction. Approximately 30% of undergraduate tanners reported neglecting responsibilities and 14% missed a day or part of a day of school or work because of tanning (Ashrafioun and Bonar, 2014b). However, only a minority (6%) of frequent tanners reported missing important activities or getting in trouble at work or with friends because of tanning (Harrington et al., 2011). This criterion is likewise one of the most severe, and least often endorsed, of the criteria for substance use and gambling disorders (Hasin et al., 2013).

Addictive behaviors often persist despite knowledge and experiences of the risks. The cancer and other health risks of excessive UVR exposure are well-established (Bataille, 2013; Colantonio et al., 2014; Wehner et al., 2012), and many tanners report an awareness of the risks but continue to tan. For example, Knight and colleagues (2002) found that more than 90% of undergraduate indoor tanning users indicated that skin cancer and premature skin aging were possible complications of tanning bed use. Nearly 90% of frequent tanners indicate they continue to tan despite knowing that it is bad for them (Harrington et al., 2011). Tanning also persists in the face of the experience of risks. Indoor tanning users and sunbathers continue to tan despite experiencing painful sunburns (Cokkinides et al., 2009; Petersen et al., 2013; Stapleton et al., 2013). A compelling report demonstrated that tanning persists even among individuals diagnosed with skin cancer (Cartmel et al., 2014). In this study, participants with a diagnosis of basal cell carcinoma and a history of indoor tanning prior to diagnosis were surveyed on their indoor tanning following diagnosis. Those with symptoms of tanning addiction were significantly more likely to tan following their diagnosis compared to those without symptoms.

These studies provide evidence that the experience of tanning addiction is similar to the experiences of other behavioral addictions. A primary limitation of this work is the lack of studies specifically designed to examine the unique adverse consequences of excessive tanning (for an exception, see Harrington et al., 2011). There is a need to study the firsthand experiences of tanners who exhibit symptoms of tanning addiction, perhaps through guided interviews or other qualitative approaches. Considerable insight could be gained by asking excessive tanners to describe the problematic aspects of tanning. In addition, the studies to date have focused primarily on adolescent and young adult college samples and do not reflect the range of experiences with older tanners, who may have more advanced tanning addictions. Given these limitations, we are not yet able to make the case that the problems associated with tanning addiction meet the criteria for the disruptive experiences of substance addiction.

METHODS FOR ASSESSMENT AND PREVALENCE RATES

The SITAD is currently the only instrument designed to address potential diagnostic criteria for tanning addiction. The SITAD is a self-administered, computer-based survey developed based on the Structured Clinical Interview for DSM-IV Axis 1 disorders for opiate use disorder (Hillhouse et al., 2012). A strength of the SITAD is the development of assessment items based on qualitative research with tanners. Tanners were asked to provide feedback on whether the items were consistent with their experiences and to provide suggestions for improvement.

The SITAD was based on DSM-IV diagnoses for substance use disorders, which provided both abuse and dependence criteria, and these criteria are now represented with a unitary structure in DSM-5. In order to be categorized as tanning dependent on the SITAD, an individual has to respond affirmatively to three or more of the following criteria: (1) feeling a loss of control of amount of tanning; (2) a desire to cut down on tanning; (3) spending a great deal of time tanning; (4) social, recreational, or occupational problems or consequences from tanning; (5) continuing to tan despite experiencing physical or psychological problems from tanning; (6) tolerance to tanning; and (7) feelings of withdrawal from tanning. A classification of tanning abuse is met when an individual does not meet three or more of the previous criteria but reports at least one of the following: (1) recurrent tanning that caused a failure to fulfill work, school, or home obligations; (2) recurrent tanning despite perceived physical harm; (3) recurrent tanning-related financial or legal problems; and (4) tanning despite related recurrent social or interpersonal problems. All SITAD items contain yes or no response options and are written in a way that can refer specifically to indoor tanning, sunbathing, or both. A full listing of the items and the scoring metric can be found elsewhere (Hillhouse et al., 2012).

The SITAD has been administered in one study of 296 undergraduate students. Results indicated that 5% met the criteria for tanning dependence, and an additional 11% were at risk. A strength of the SITAD includes the demonstration of some aspects of validity and reliability. Nearly 75% of the participants identified as tanning dependent on the SITAD reported using indoor tanning at least once a week throughout the entire year. Participants identified as tanning dependent on the SITAD reported indoor tanning nearly 10 times more often during a 6-month period compared to participants with no SITAD diagnosis. Furthermore, the 6-month test–retest reliability of the SITAD was high. However, the SITAD is based on DSM-IV abuse and dependence criteria that are now combined in a unitary structure in DSM-5. Additional changes in the DSM-5 included the removal of the criterion for committing illegal acts, the addition of a criterion for craving, and the reduction of the threshold for diagnosis to meeting 2 or more of 11 criteria. Future work with the SITAD should evaluate whether similar symptoms and this new cut-point are reliable and valid in assessing tanning addictions in the context of the DSM-5 substance use disorder criteria.

Screening instruments for tanning addiction have also been developed, primarily by adapting existing alcohol screening assessments or using survey items based on DSM-IV substance abuse criteria (Warthan et al., 2005). By definition, screening questionnaires are expected to yield high rates of false positives because a positive screen would need to be followed by a more formal assessment for diagnostic purposes. These assessments and related adaptations, referred to as the mCAGE (modified CAGE) and mDSM-IV (modified DSM-IV) (Warthan et al., 2005), have become the most commonly used assessments of tanning addiction. The mCAGE is a tanning adapted version of the four-item CAGE (Cut down, Annoyed, Guilty, Eye-opener) assessment for problematic alcohol use. The mDSM-IV was developed based on the diagnostic criteria for substance abuse and dependence outlined in the DSM-IV text revision (DSM-IV-TR). These criteria include tolerance (needing increased amounts of exposure to get desired effect), withdrawal (irritability or restlessness when exposure is less than desired), greater exposure than one intended, desire and attempts to reduce amount of use, a great deal of effortful behavior to get exposure, reduced involvement in social and other activities because of use, and continued use despite problems likely caused or made worse by exposure. The mDSM-IV consists of a seven-question survey scale.

The mCAGE and mDSM-IV have raised awareness that tanners experience aspects of tanning addiction. Unfortunately, there is little published information about the psychometric properties of these screening assessments (with the exception of Heckman et al., 2014b), and fundamental questions remain about their validity. One problem is the unusually high prevalence rates of tanning addiction symptoms found with these screeners. Tanning addiction rates among general samples that include both tanners and non-tanners have ranged from 11% to 53% based on the mCAGE and mDSM-IV (Harrington et al., 2011; Heckman et al., 2008, 2014a; Mosher and Danoff-Burg, 2010; Poorsattar and Hornung, 2007; Warthan et al., 2005). A study by Schneider and colleagues (2014) demonstrated serious concerns about the validity of the mCAGE. The researchers interviewed tanners and found a wide range of interpretations of the meaning of the items. In addition, scores on the mCAGE did not correspond with excessive tanning behavior. Nearly 57% of tanning bed users identified as tanning addicted on the mCAGE had not visited a tanning salon in the previous week, with 38% reporting no tanning in the previous month.

It is difficult to estimate the prevalence of tanning addition given the limitations with commonly used screening assessments. It is also preliminary to estimate such rates given the lack of accepted and validated criteria for tanning addiction. Both tanning addiction screening and diagnostic assessments are needed that accurately represent the physiological and psychological symptoms that define tanning addiction rather than relying exclusively on adapting criteria for substance use disorders. Phenomenological studies of the experiences of tanning addiction could be useful in the development of such measures. We recently developed and evaluated an alternative screening approach informed by behavioral models of addiction (Stapleton et al., submitted for publication). The seven-item Behavioral Addiction Indoor Tanning Screener (BAITS) assesses symptoms of behavioral addiction to tanning that include feelings of diminished control over tanning as well as urges and cravings to engage in tanning. We established scoring criteria for the BAITS and found that 9% of ever users of indoor tanning scored positively for multiple symptoms of tanning addiction. Tanners identified as symptomatic of tanning addiction on the BAITS reported nearly five times more indoor tanning sessions in the following 6 months compared to other tanners. In addition, nearly 75% of individuals identified by the BAITS as symptomatic were identified as tanning dependent on the SITAD.

COMORBIDITIES

Studies of the correlates of tanning addiction have included measures of substance use and psychiatric conditions. The presence of tanning addiction and these comorbidities may suggest a shared physiopathology. However, it is important to consider that studies related to the comorbidities of tanning addiction are based on associations with the mCAGE or mDSM-IV. The aforementioned limitations of these assessments mean that observed associations should be interpreted with caution.

Substance Use

If tanning is an addiction, in theory it should be related to other addictions. A full understanding of the association between tanning addiction and substance use and other addictive disorders is lacking due in large part to the lack of consensus on classifying tanning addiction. Nevertheless, some studies have found increased rates of at least some substance use disorders or problems and tanning addiction. Participants who screened positively for tanning addiction reported a greater number of alcohol use days (Mosher and Danoff-Burg, 2010) and were more likely to report at least one symptom of alcohol abuse or dependence (Heckman et al., 2014a) compared to participants who did not screen positive. Ashrafioun and Bonar (2014a) found that hazardous drinking was positively associated with mDSM-IV, but not mCAGE, classifications of tanning addiction. The association with tobacco use and tanning dependence is not consistent. Heckman and colleagues (2008) found that those with tanning addictive symptoms were more likely to report smoking in the past 30 days compared to others. However, subsequent studies of tanners have not found associations with smoking and measures of tanning addiction (Harrington et al., 2011; Heckman et al., 2014a; Mosher and Danoff-Burg, 2010; Zeller et al., 2006). Weak and inconsistent associations have been observed with tanning addiction and marijuana and other illicit drug use as well (Ashrafioun and Bonar, 2014b; Harrington et al., 2011; Heckman et al., 2014a; Mosher and Danoff-Burg, 2010). Thus, the extent to which tanning addiction and substance use disorders co-occur is unclear.

Other Psychiatric Conditions

Few studies have examined the association of other psychiatric conditions with tanning addiction, and the observed associations have not been consistent across studies. Heckman and colleagues (2014a) administered the Mini International Neuropsychiatric Interview (MINI), an assessment for a variety of psychiatric conditions, to a sample of 306 undergraduate females. The authors found little evidence of differences between those who screened positive for tanning addiction and those who did not on the endorsement of symptoms of other psychiatric conditions, including eating disorders, depression, social anxiety, post-traumatic stress, or generalized anxiety. Harrington and colleagues (2011) found no association between tanning addiction and screening assessments for anxiety, schizophrenia, and bipolar disorder. No association has been observed between screening measures of general depression symptoms and tanning addiction (Ashrafioun and Bonar, 2014a; Harrington et al., 2011; Heckman et al., 2014a; Mosher and Danoff-Burg, 2010).

Heckman and colleagues (2014a) found that scores on screening measures of tanning addiction were associated with symptoms of seasonal affective disorder (SAD). Hillhouse and colleagues (2005) found that frequent indoor tanning users (defined as using indoor tanning 40 or more times in the previous year) were more likely to report symptoms of SAD compared to less frequent tanners. SAD is a seasonal pattern of depression thought to be caused by alterations in serotonin and melatonin, hormones that regulate sleep patterns and mood. SAD is often treated with light therapy in order to modify irregular circadian rhythms. The alteration of serotonin levels by UVR exposure is an alternative explanation for excessive tanning behavior (for review, see Kourosh et al., 2010). Specifically, UVR inhibits the conversion of serotonin, which is involved in brain pleasure pathways, to melatonin. Wehr and colleagues' (2001) research suggests that individuals suffering from SAD experience an overproduction of melatonin during winter months. Tanners with SAD symptoms may be self-medicating with UVR, which may increase serotonin levels by inhibiting the conversion to melatonin and thereby help in the regulation of sleep and mood (Hillhouse et al., 2005).

Some investigators have suggested that excessive tanning may be a specific manifestation of body dysmorphic disorder (BDD). Tanning BDD has been shown to manifest in individuals with BDD through an obsession with modifying one's natural and unsatisfactory skin color, which leads to a compulsive desire for tanning (Phillips et al., 2006). Case studies describe a high prevalence of BDD symptoms in dermatology patients with a history of tanning (Hunter-Yates et al., 2007). The view of excessive tanning as a compulsive behavior suggests that tanning would not be pleasurable but, rather, serves as relief from discomfort caused by an obsessive need to tan to correct a perceived image problem. In contrast, an endogenous opioid model of tanning addiction assumes that tanning may relate more to an impulsive or addictive behavior motivated by the pleasure and mood boost gained from tanning, which ultimately may also result in physiological dependence symptoms that further drive the behavior. Future biological and psychological research may provide insights into whether excessive tanning is better aligned with substance use and behavioral addictions, SAD, or BDD.

RISK AND PROTECTIVE FACTORS

A number of studies have examined tanning addiction risk and protective factors. Because these studies based their categorization of addiction on the mCAGE and mDSM-IV, the results again should be interpreted with caution.

Demographic Factors

Female tanners are more likely to screen positive for tanning addiction compared to male tanners (Ashrafioun and Bonar, 2014a; Harrington et al., 2011; Mosher and Danoff-Burg, 2010; Poorsattar and Hornung,

2007; Zeller et al., 2006). A younger age of initiation of tanning is related to a higher likelihood of reporting tanning addiction (Harrington et al., 2011; Zeller et al., 2006). Studies have not, however, found an association between age at assessment and tanning addiction (Ashrafioun and Bonar, 2014a; Mosher and Danoff-Burg, 2010; Warthan et al., 2005). Most of these studies involve adolescent and young adult samples and thus focus on a limited age range. Participants in these samples are also primarily white, and many are university students. This makes it difficult to assess the association of tanning addiction with socioeconomic status, race, and other demographic factors.

Genetics

There is a dearth of studies regarding possible genetic underpinnings of tanning addiction. In a notable recent study, Cartmel and colleagues (2014) reported on the first exome-wide association study of tanning addiction. The authors compared genetic expression in 79 participants with symptoms of tanning addiction with 213 tanners not classified as tanning addicted. The exome-wide analysis found that significantly fewer participants classified as tanning addicted had a minor allele in one gene, patched domain containing 2 (*PTCHD2*), compared to non-tanning addicted participants. The primary function of *PTCHD2* is unknown. Cartmel and colleagues also conducted a candidate gene analysis of genes known to be associated with substance dependence. They found additional genetic differences in candidate genes in three of four single nucleotide polymorphisms (SNPs) within the ankyrin repeat and kinase domain containing 1 (*ANKK1*) gene. The associations were not significant after Bonferroni corrections on the significance level criterion. However, these findings are consistent with work by Flores and colleagues (2013), who examined the association of indoor tanning and SNPs in genes implicated in dopamine regulation and drug metabolism. The authors did not include a measure of tanning addiction but, rather, compared participants who ever used indoor tanning with participants who never used indoor tanning. They found variants in SNPs in *DRD2* and *ANKK1* genes associated with ever use of indoor tanning. These genes are involved with dopamine receptors and signaling pathways. Although some preliminary findings suggest a potential genetic component to tanning addiction, clearly much more research is needed to better understand these initial associations.

TREATMENTS

Few interventions have been designed specifically for tanning addiction or for frequent tanners. There is evidence that a brief in-person intervention can be efficacious in reducing tanning among frequent tanners, defined as using indoor tanning 10 or more times in the previous year. Turrisi and colleagues (2008) tested a peer-delivered motivational interviewing (MI) intervention in a sample of 39 female undergraduates. The goal of the 30-minute MI peer counseling session was to provide participants with cognitive behavioral skills information and to encourage participants to evaluate the effects of their indoor tanning behavior. MI participants reported significantly fewer indoor tanning sessions compared to control participants during the 3 months following the intervention. Tanning addiction status was not reported in this study. Future studies are needed to evaluate more carefully the efficacy of motivational and other therapeutic approaches to treating tanning addiction in larger samples and with more extensive follow-up periods.

FUTURE DIRECTIONS

Tanning addiction is an important issue with implications for the mental health as well as public health fields given the associated risk for skin cancer. There is compelling but preliminary evidence that tanning addiction shares features expected in models of behavioral addiction. The strongest evidence for tanning addiction comes from lab and mouse studies that demonstrate a biological reward pathway of UVR exposure. This work provides evidence that endogenous opioids may be implicated in tanning addiction. Human studies show that frequent tanners can differentiate between UVR-emitting tanning beds and sham beds and respond to the administration of an opioid blocking drug, in a manner that is somewhat similar to those with opioid use disorders. The demonstration that tanning activates biological reward pathways and may influence physiology is critically important for moving toward classifying and understanding the pathophysiology of the condition, as well as developing efficacious methods for prevention and treatment. Addiction also requires persistent behavioral urges that result in compulsive and disruptive behaviors. There is some evidence of the personally problematic nature of tanning addiction, although studies are needed to capture the unique experiences of tanning addiction.

As a whole, the evidence regarding tanning addiction is not yet sufficient to support an official recognition of tanning as a psychiatric disorder, behavioral addiction or otherwise. The evidence does, however, provide some preliminary support for the consideration of tanning as a behavior with addictive potential and supports the need for further research efforts. We have proposed criteria for tanning addiction and provided the published literature that supports these criteria. Additional work is needed to support this conceptualization of tanning addiction and provide insights into adapting symptoms into formal diagnostic criteria.

Research is needed to quantify the amount of tanning behavior associated with tanning addiction. It is often inferred that some individuals tan far more than necessary to maintain cosmetic benefits, but it is difficult to create an empirically derived rate of tanning that would be considered excessive. Many authors consider frequent tanning to be use of indoor tanning more than 10 times in a year (e.g., Demko et al., 2003; Guy et al., 2014). This definition is valuable from a public health perspective because the risk for skin cancer from indoor tanning use is exponentially increased at this rate (Cust et al., 2011; Lazovich et al., 2010). However, this definition is less helpful with tanning addiction because someone with a tanning addiction would likely tan regularly throughout the year. In the UVR sham tanning bed experimental studies, frequent tanners were defined as participants who used tanning beds at least 8 to 15 times per month (Feldman et al., 2004). Hillhouse and colleagues (2007) examined patterns of indoor tanning behavior and found a subset of "regular" tanners, 12% of all tanners, who were likely to report use of indoor tanning throughout the year and tanning in response to negative mood. Much less is known about frequent outdoor tanning. It is likely that year-round tanners in temperate climates would exhibit seasonal variations in use of indoor tanning when outdoor tanning is not feasible in cold weather. Phenomenological studies with those who tan multiple times per week are likely to provide valuable insights related to quantifying excessive tanning behaviors and screening for tanning addiction. Although the diagnosis of substance use disorders similarly does not include frequency criteria, frequency variables related to tanning may provide valuable information for evaluating or screening for tanning addiction, and they will also indicate ranges at which clinically significant problems begin to manifest.

There is only modest evidence that individuals can have urges or cravings to tan, or that excessive tanning can interfere in a clinically significant manner with daily functioning or cause interpersonal, social, or professional problems. These are hallmarks of behavioral addictions. The substance abuse literature contains valuable examples of phenomenological studies with individuals suffering from addiction that provide rich experiential details about the addiction process (e.g., Grant et al., 2010). Similar studies with tanners could advance our understanding of the experiences of excessive tanners and provide a detailed phenomenological account of tanning addiction. This may include their current tanning behavior, their lifetime history of tanning, and the developmental course of their tanning addiction, as well as the expression of adverse consequences. More research is needed to identify the types and extent of adverse consequences from excessive tanning, which may differ vastly from those related to substance use disorders or other behavioral addictions.

Once the adverse consequences of excessive tanning are better understood, instruments that reliably and validly assess the condition can be developed and tested. The existing screening instruments, primarily created through adapting screening assessments for substance use disorders, lack strong psychometric properties, and they identify rates of tanning addiction that are extraordinarily high. A preferable approach is to create assessments with items designed specifically to capture the unique perspectives and experiences of excessive tanners. With one notable exception (Hillhouse et al., 2012), preliminary qualitative research with tanners was not reported in the development of these assessments. The SITAD is the only proposed "diagnostic" assessment of tanning addiction, but more work is needed to determine whether tanning addiction constitutes a unique psychiatric disorder and ascertain appropriate diagnostic criteria. Validated measures of tanning addiction will be critically important to conducting behavioral, experimental, or genetic studies to better understand the condition.

Additional evidence of the physiological effects of tanning addiction is needed to establish whether tanning addiction is similar in key ways to substance addiction. Harrington and colleagues' (2012) SPECT study provided the first evidence that central neural dopamine pathways are activated through UVR exposure. Magnetic resonance imaging (MRI) could be a useful method for examining the physiological changes that may occur in the brain due to tanning (Nolan and Feldman, 2009). For example, functional MRIs could be used to demonstrate that tanning-related stimuli, such as the smell of tanning lotions or images of tanning beds, results in activation of pleasure centers in the brain. It would also be informative to ascertain whether imaging studies of those with tanning addiction and substance use disorders or other behavioral addictions have similar differences relative to controls in terms of structural differences in brain regions and in the quantity of dopamine receptors in the brain. Positron emission tomography could be used to demonstrate the role of dopamine and dopamine receptors in the physiological response to UVR exposure.

Implications of Tanning Addiction for Treatments and Policy

The preliminary evidence regarding tanning addiction is sufficiently compelling that it highlights the need to raise public awareness about the addictive potential of tanning. Mental health professionals should remain open to the possibility that tanning may be addictive and consider providing counseling to excessive tanners related to their behavior. Tanning addiction may be reduced by brief intervention approaches such as MI alone, or it may require more intensive interventions including cognitive behavioral, supportive, or other therapy. It is likely that tanners with tanning addiction may be resistant to change. The MI approach is designed to promote behavioral change talk among resistant individuals through sympathetic and empathic counseling techniques (Hettema et al., 2005). MI interventions encourage participants to work through ambivalence about their need to reduce their tanning behavior and to encourage change talk regarding the desirability, reasons, or need to change their tanning behaviors (Hettema et al., 2005). MI approaches have shown some preliminary evidence of efficacy in the indoor tanning literature (Heckman et al., 2013; Turrisi et al. 2008), although larger-scale and longer-term trials with excessive tanners are needed.

Finally, tanning addiction research supports the need for increased legislation and regulation of indoor tanning among adolescents. Many adolescents engage in indoor tanning, and this developmental period is marked by ongoing brain development. Adolescents are particularly vulnerable to the effects of potentially addictive exposures. Legal restrictions for substances with associated health risks, such as tobacco products and alcoholic beverages, are widely used governmental strategies to restrict access by underage populations. Laws that restrict or ban minors from using indoor tanning have been enacted or are being considered in several U.S. states.

Conclusion

The evidence for tanning addiction is sufficient to suggest that tanning exhibits important features of a behavioral addiction. There is a plausible biological reward pathway of UVR exposure and some evidence of problematic aspects of tanning addiction. However, more research is warranted to expand our understanding of the physiology and experience of tanning addiction in order to evaluate its potential status as a psychiatric condition.

REFERENCES

American Psychiatric Association, 2013. Diagnostic and statistical manual of mental disorders (fifth ed.). Washington, DC: American Psychiatric Association.

Ashrafioun, L., Bonar, E.E., 2014a. Tanning addiction and psychopathology: Further evaluation of anxiety disorders and substance abuse. J Am Acad Dermatol. 70, 473–480.

Ashrafioun, L., Bonar, E.E., 2014b. Development of a brief scale to assess frequency of symptoms and problems associated with tanning. J Am Acad Dermatol. 70, 588–589.

Bataille, V., 2013. Sunbed use increases risk of melanoma; Risk increases with greater number of sessions and first use at younger age. Evid Based Nurs. 16, 107–108.

Cartmel, B., Dewan, A., Ferrucci, L.M., Gelernter, J., Stapleton, J.L., Mayne, S.T., et al., 2014. Novel gene identified in a genome-wide association study of tanning dependence. Exp Dermatol. 23(10), 757–759.

Chan, A., 2012, May 3. Patricia Krentcil, "tanning mom," bringing attention to "tanorexia": How dangerous is it? Retrieved August 26, 2014, from http://www.huffingtonpost.com/2012/05/03/patricia-krentcil-tanning-mom-tanorexia_n_1475138.html

Cokkinides, V., Weinstock, M., Lazovich, D., Ward, E., Thun, M., 2009. Indoor tanning use among adolescents in the U.S., 1998 to 2004. Cancer. 115, 190–198.

Colantonio, S., Bracken, M.B., Beecker, J., 2014. The association of indoor tanning and melanoma in adults: Systematic review and meta-analysis. J Am Acad Dermatol. 70, 847–857.

Cui, R., Widlund, H.R., Feige, E., Lin, J.Y., Wilensky, D.L., Igras, V.E., et al., 2007. Central role of p53 in the suntan response and pathologic hyperpigmentation. Cell. 128, 853–864.

Cust, A.E., Armstrong, B.K., Goumas, C., Jenkins, M.A., Schmid, H., Hopper, J.L., et al. 2011. Sunbed use during adolescence and early adulthood is associated with increased risk of early-onset melanoma. Int J Cancer. 128, 2425–2435.

Davis, L., Riley, D., 2012, May 3. "Tanning Mom": Does New Jersey woman suffer from "tanerexia"? Retrieved August 26, 2014, from http://abcnews.go.com/US/tanning-mom-jersey-woman-suffer-tanorexia/story?id=16267543

Demko, C.A., Borawski, E.A., Debanne, S.M., Cooper, K.D., Stange, K.C., 2003. Use of indoor tanning facilities by white adolescents in the United States. Arch Pediatr Adolesc Med. 157, 854–860.

Feldman, S.R., Liguori, A., Kucenic, M., Rapp, S.R., Fleischer, A.B., Jr., Lang, W., et al., 2004. Ultraviolet exposure is a reinforcing stimulus in frequent indoor tanners. J Am Acad Dermatol. 51, 45–51.

Fell, G.L., Robinson, K.C., Mao, J., Woolf, C.J., Fisher, D.E., 2014. Skin β-endorphin mediates addiction to UV light. Cell. 157, 1527–1534.

Flores, K.G., Erdei, E., Luo, L., White, K.A., Leng, S., Berwick, M., et al., 2013. A pilot study of genetic variants in dopamine regulators with indoor tanning and melanoma. Exp Dermatol. 22, 576–581.

Gambichler, T., Bader, A., Vojvodic, M., Avermaete, A., Schenk, M., Altmeyer, P., et al., 2002. Plasma levels of opioid peptides after sunbed exposures. Br J Dermatol. 147, 1207–1211.

Gilchrest, B.A., Park, H.Y., Eller, M.S., Yaar, M., 1996. Mechanisms of ultraviolet light-induced pigmentation. Photochem Photobiol. 63, 1–10.

Grant, J.E., Potenza, M.N., Weinstein, A., Gorelick, D.A., 2010. Introduction to behavioral addictions. Am J Drug Alcohol Abuse. 36, 233–241.

Guy, G.P., Berkowitz, Z., Tai, E., Holman, D.M., Jones, S.E., Richardson, L.C., 2014. Indoor tanning among high school students in the United States, 2009 and 2011. JAMA Dermatol. 150, 501–511.

Harrington, C.R., Beswick, T.C., Leitenberger, J., Minhajuddin, A., Jacobe, H.T., Adinoff, B., 2011. Addictive-like behaviours to ultraviolet light among frequent indoor tanners. Clin Exp Dermatol. 36, 33–38.

Harrington, C.R., Beswick, T.C., Graves, M., Jacobe, H.T., Harris, T.S., Kourosh, S., et al., 2012. Activation of the mesostriatal reward pathway with exposure to ultraviolet radiation (UVR) vs. sham UVR in frequent tanners: A pilot study. Addict Biol. 17, 680–686.

Hasin, D.S., O'Brien, C.P., Auriacombe, M., Borges, G., Bucholz, K., Budney, A., et al., 2013. DSM-5 criteria for substance use disorders: Recommendations and rationale. Am J Psychiatry. 170, 834–851.

Heckman, C.J., Egleston, B.L., Wilson, D.B., Ingersoll, K.S., 2008. A preliminary investigation of the predictors of tanning dependence. Am J Health Behav. 32, 451–464.

Heckman, C.J., Zhu, F., Manne, S.L., Kloss, J.D., Collins, B.N., Bass, S.B., et al., 2013. Process and outcomes of a skin protection intervention for young adults. J Health Psychol. 18, 561–573.

Heckman, C.J., Cohen-Filipic, J., Darlow, S., Kloss, J.D., Manne, S.L., Munshi, T., 2014a. Psychiatric and addictive symptoms of young adult female indoor tanners. Am J Health Promot. 28, 168–174.

Heckman, C.J., Darlow, S., Kloss, J.D., Cohen-Filipic, J., Manne, S.L., Munshi, T., et al., 2014b. Measurement of tanning dependence. J Eur Acad Dermatol Venereol. 28, 1179–1185.

Hettema, J., Steele, J., Miller, W.R., 2005. Motivational interviewing. Annu Rev Clin Psychol. 1, 91–111.

Hillhouse, J., Stapleton, J., Turrisi, R., 2005. Association of frequent indoor UV tanning with seasonal affective disorder. Arch Dermatol. 141, 1465–1465.

Hillhouse, J., Turrisi, R., Shields, A.L., 2007. Patterns of indoor tanning use: Implications for clinical interventions. Arch Dermatol. 143, 1530–1535.

Hillhouse, J.J., Baker, M.K., Turrisi, R., Shields, A., Stapleton, J., Jain, S., et al., 2012. Evaluating a measure of tanning abuse and dependence. Arch Dermatol. 148, 815–819.

Hunter-Yates, J., Dufresne, R.G., Phillips, K.A., 2007. Tanning in body dsymorphic disorder. J Am Acad Dermatol. 56, S107–S109.

Kaur, M., Feldman, S.R., Liguori, A., Fleischer, A.B., 2005. Indoor tanning relieves pain. Photodermatol Photoimmunol Photomed. 21, 278–278.

Kaur, M., Liguori, A., Fleischer, A.B., Jr., Feldman, S.R., 2006. Plasma beta-endorphin levels in frequent and infrequent tanners before and after ultraviolet and non-ultraviolet stimuli. J Am Acad Dermatol. 54, 919–920.

Knight, J.M., Kirincich, A.N., Farmer, E.R., Hood, A.F., 2002. Awareness of the risks of tanning lamps does not influence behavior among college students. Arch Dermatol. 138, 1311–1315.

Kourosh, A.S., Harrington, C.R., Adinoff, B., 2010. Tanning as a behavioral addiction. Am J Drug Alcohol Abuse. 36, 284–290.

Lazovich, D., Vogel, R.I., Berwick, M., Weinstock, M.A., Anderson, K.E., Warshaw, E.M., 2010. Indoor tanning and risk of melanoma: A case–control study in a highly exposed population. Cancer Epidemiol Biomarkers Prev. 19, 1557–1568.

Levins, P., Carr, D., Fisher, J., Momtaz, K., Parrish, J., 1983. Plasma β-endorphin and β-lipotropin response to ultraviolet radiation. Lancet. 322, 166.

Mosher, C.E., Danoff-Burg, S., 2010. Addiction to indoor tanning: Relation to anxiety, depression, and substance use. Arch Dermatol. 146, 412–417.

Nolan, B.V., Feldman, S.R., 2009. Ultraviolet tanning addiction. Dermatol Clin. 27, 109–112.

Petersen, B., Thieden, E., Philipsen, P.A., Heydenreich, J., Young, A.R., Wulf, H.C., 2013. A sun holiday is a sunburn holiday. Photodermatol Photoimmunol Photomed. 29, 221–224.

Phillips, K.A., Conroy, M., Dufresne, R.G., Menard, W., Didie, E.R., Hunter-Yates, J., et al., 2006. Tanning in body dysmorphic disorder. Psychiatr Q. 77, 129–138.

Poorsattar, S.P., Hornung, R.L., 2007. UV light abuse and high-risk tanning behavior among undergraduate college students. J Am Acad Dermatol. 56, 375–379.

Roth-Deri, I., Green-Sadan, T., Yadid, G., 2008. Beta-endorphin and drug-induced reward and reinforcement. Prog Neurobiol. 86, 1–21.

Schauer, E., Trautinger, F., Köck, A., Schwarz, A., Bhardwaj, R., Simon, M., et al., 1994. Proopiomelanocortin-derived peptides are synthesized and released by human keratinocytes. J Clin Invest. 93, 2258.

Schneider, S., Schirmbeck, F., Bock, C., Greinert, R., Breitbart, E.W., Diehl, K., 2014. Casting shadows on the prevalence of tanning dependence: An assessment of mCAGE criteria. Acta Derm Venereol. 95(2), 162–168.

Shah, A., Smith, S., Heckman, C.J., Feldman, S.R., 2012. Tanning dependence: Is tanning an addiction? In: Heckman, C.J., Manne, S.L. (Eds.), Shedding light on indoor tanning (pp. 107–120). Dordrecht, The Netherlands" Springer.

Stapleton, J.L., Hillhouse, J., Turrisi, R., Robinson, J.K., Baker, K., Manne, S.L., et al., 2013. Erythema and ultraviolet indoor tanning: Findings from a diary study. Transl Behav Med. 3, 10–16.

Stapleton, J.L., Hillhouse, J., Turrisi, R., Baker, K., Manne, S.L., Coups, E.J., 2014. The Behavioral Addiction Indoor Tanning Screener (BAITITS): An evaluation of a brief measure of behavioral addictive syptoms. Manuscript submitted for publication.

Turrisi, R., Mastroleo, N.R., Stapleton, J., Mallett, K., 2008. A comparison of two brief intervention approaches to reduce indoor tanning behavior in young women who indoor tan very frequently. Arch Dermatol. 144, 1521–1524.

Warthan, M.M., Uchida, T., Wagner, R.F., 2005. UV light tanning as a type of substance-related disorder. Arch Dermatol. 141, 963–966.

Wehner, M.R., Shive, M.L., Chren, M.M., Han, J., Qureshi, A.A., Linos, E., 2012. Indoor tanning and non-melanoma skin cancer: Systematic review and meta-analysis. BMJ. 345, e5909.

Wehr, T.A., Duncan, W.C., Jr, Sher, L., Aeschbach, D., Schwartz, P.J., Turner, E.H., Postolache, T.T., Rosenthal, N.E. 2001. A circadian signal of change of season in patients with seasonal affective disorder. Arch Gen Psychiatry. 58(12), 1108–1114.

Wintzen, M., Ostijn, D.M., Polderman, M.C., Le Cessie, S., Burbach, J.P.H., Vermeer, B.J., 2001. Total body exposure to ultraviolet radiation does not influence plasma levels of immunoreactive β-endorphin in man. Photodermatol Photoimmunol Photomed. 17, 256–260.

Zeller, S., Lazovich, D., Forster, J., Widome, R., 2006. Do adolescent indoor tanners exhibit dependency? J Am Acad Dermatol. 54, 589–596.

10

Conclusions and Future Directions to Advance the Science and Clinical Care of Behavioral Addictions

NANCY M. PETRY ■

This book describes research related to non-substance behavioral addictions, including gambling, gaming, Internet use, sexual behaviors, shopping, exercising, eating, and tanning. Although the fifth edition of the *Diagnostic and Statistical Manual of Mental Disorders* (DSM-5; American Psychiatric Association, 2013) officially recognizes only one of these conditions (i.e., gambling), the others have varying degrees of evidence related to their diagnosis, prevalence rates, neurophysiology, and treatment. As science progresses, future medical classification systems may include some of these conditions.

Early psychiatric diagnostic systems relied relatively little on empirical data, but as psychiatric diagnosis and treatment are advancing, the current systems are requiring evidence of reliability and validity of diagnosis. For example, when the DSM-III initially included pathological gambling in 1980, very little research existed regarding classification or expression of this disorder. Clinicians and society recognized that excessive gambling could cause harms, but no widely accepted criteria were available. The DSM-III allowed criteria based on clinical experiences alone. The prevalence rate of the condition was unknown at that time, and its neurobiological underpinnings were almost entirely unstudied. Leisure and Blume (1987) developed the first widely applied screening instrument, The South Oaks Gambling Screen, years after the DSM-III initially introduced excessive gambling as a psychiatric disorder. Treatment for gambling occurred in only a handful of specialized centers, and no large-scale randomized trials of interventions existed until the 21st century.

During the past 15 years, the scientific research on gambling disorder has burgeoned. As Chapter 2 describes, there are now dozens of controlled trials of treatments, scores of neurobiological and genetics studies, and large-scale epidemiological surveys assessing prevalence rates in countries throughout the world. Substantial evidence exists that gambling disorder overlaps with substance use disorders in terms of phenomenology, comorbidity, risk factors and natural history, and genetics and neurobiology. The progression of research on gambling disorder should be a model for scientific investigation of other putative behavioral addictions. When DSM-6 is in its formative stages, the inclusion of other behavioral addictions as psychiatric conditions will require data similar to those now available related to gambling disorder.

As Dr. Rehbein and colleagues describe in Chapter 3, research on Internet gaming disorder is progressing at a rapid pace. This is the only behavioral addiction included in the research appendix of the DSM-5. As scientists, clinicians, and the public are gaining awareness of difficulties that can arise from excessive game playing behaviors, researchers are coming to a consensus in terms of defining this condition. Recently, key articles have outlined criteria that embody the condition, but the operationalization of these criteria must be tested empirically across multiple populations and contexts. It is now clear that this condition should only refer to individuals who have suffered clinically significant harms from their game playing behaviors, as opposed to persons who simply spend a lot of time playing or who occasionally lose sleep from playing games too late at night without any significant adverse consequences. Nevertheless, the unique nature and course of problems that arise from excessive gaming playing behaviors require additional investigation. They may vary cross culturally and by developmental stage. They may also be transient, and if so, this information may preclude inclusion of this condition as a psychiatric disorder. More longitudinal studies must evaluate the natural history of the condition to better understand its clinical significance and prognosis. Only limited data exist regarding prevalence rates of Internet gaming disorder in general populations, and the majority of studies are limited to youth and young adults. Although specialized treatment facilities exist, there are very little data on the efficacy or effectiveness of interventions.

Importantly, the DSM-5 text states that Internet gaming addiction refers to problems associated with playing *any* type of electronic games. People can develop problems with online and offline games, as well as with games played on handheld devices and gaming consoles. The title of the condition contains the term "Internet" because this is the venue through which most persons are currently experiencing problems with gaming. It was also included to distinguish the name of this condition from "gambling disorder," which is likely to be confused with the phrase "gaming disorder." Future research on Internet gaming disorder will need to ascertain whether the difficulties that arise from different gaming formats are similar conceptually. As technology continues to progress, new games will emerge, and it is important that criteria developed and empirically tested are broad enough to capture persons who experience clinically significant difficulties with multiple formats and presentations of electronic games. Studies evaluating the neurobiological basis of this condition are also critical to its eventual classification as a psychiatric disorder. As psychiatric diagnosis becomes more objective and moves toward biological indices when possible, results from biologically based studies ultimately may serve to distinguish Internet gaming disorder from other conditions and to evaluate its potential similarities and differences with other non-substance addictive disorders and other related conditions as well.

Drs. Rumpf and colleagues outline the controversy surrounding Internet addiction more globally in Chapter 4. Clearly, the proportion of the population that exhibits difficulties with any online activity is going to be larger than the proportion whose problems are restricted to a single online activity—that is, gaming. However, many current studies of Internet addiction report highly variable prevalence rates, with some noting that up to 50% of individuals surveyed experience problems with excessive Internet use. This rate is highly skeptical and draws into question the legitimacy of the assessment methods. Furthermore, most persons who report difficulties with excessive online behaviors have a preferred use of the Internet. Some shop excessively online, some view pornography, some play games, some gamble, and some surf the Internet or communicate with others using social media. Demographic characteristics vary markedly across persons who spend excessive amounts of time engaged in these various Internet activities. Moreover, comorbidities with other psychiatric conditions likely vary depending on the problematic Internet activity, and risk factors for and expressions of problems probably differ as well. It is not clear if Internet addiction has an underlying unitary construct or if it represents a distinct mental condition, unique from other psychiatric conditions.

Until this condition is more clearly defined, cross-study comparisons cannot be made, and estimates of prevalence rates will remain elusive. The criteria proposed for Internet gaming disorder in DSM-5 may represent an initial effort in more consistently capturing the broader condition of Internet addiction and ensuring that the criteria are tapping clinically significant harms, as opposed to simply spending excessive amounts of time online. Future investigations must also distinguish unique aspects of Internet addiction relative to those that involve excessive behaviors in related domains. For example, problems arising from excessive online gambling are likely more consistent with gambling disorder than with Internet addiction more globally. One can make a similar argument toward excessive pornography viewing and sex addiction and also excessive online shopping and compulsive shopping. Until these and related issues are resolved, mental health professionals will be unlikely to recognize Internet addiction as an independent and unique construct.

The Sexual Disorders Workgroup convened by the American Psychiatric Association proposed a disorder related to excessive sexual activities and problems arising from them. Indeed, the DSM-5 field trials included an assessment of this condition using a set of criteria that evidenced adequate reliability and validity in that sample. However, excessive sexual behaviors may represent a sexual disorder more so than an addictive disorder; these behaviors may also reflect the extreme end of a normal behavioral pattern. In Chapter 5, Drs. Campbell and Stein articulate the controversies surrounding excessive sexual behaviors and their classification. Relatively little is known about the prevalence rate of this condition in general populations, and most existing studies are limited to small clinical samples. Even less is known about its neurobiology and treatment, pharmacological or psychosocial. Several theoretical models attempt to explain this condition, but each model applies different terminology and assessment tools, making it difficult to compare across studies. Nevertheless, a clinical population exists for which high frequency and intensity sexual behaviors lead to significant distress and impairment in life functioning. Consensus on the terminology and defining features of this condition, and their associations with other psychiatric conditions generally and sexual disorders and behavioral addictions specifically, could guide clinical research to improve prevention and treatment for those experiencing distress from excessive sexual behaviors.

A fairly extensive literature exists on excessive shopping and the problems that can arise from it. As Dr. Black details in Chapter 6, several methods exist for identifying compulsive or addictive shopping, but large population studies have not yet evaluated their reliability and validity. Excessive shopping may be aligned with behavioral addictions, impulsive disorders, or compulsive disorders. Although a few large-scale epidemiological studies exist, they used different methods of classification and yielded somewhat discrepant prevalence rates. Women appear most affected in the vast majority of, but not all, studies, raising additional questions about the optimal classification of this condition and its overlap with behavioral addictions, which generally affect higher proportions of males than females. Additional studies on comorbidities of excessive shopping may confirm its relationship with other psychiatric disorders. Neurobiological and genetic studies would also help clarify these associations. More research along each of these domains may ultimately result in the inclusion of this condition as a formal psychiatric diagnosis, under the rubric of substance use and related addictions, obsessive–compulsive disorders, or impulse control disorders more broadly.

Exercising, and exercising to excess in particular, engenders biological changes including release of endorphins, as Drs. Weinstein and Weinstein outline in Chapter 7. Because of their role in substance use disorders, endogenous opioids released during excessive exercising may exert reinforcing effects, akin to those in substance use disorders. Furthermore, at least some biological evidence exists that exercising over extended periods of time, and the related release of endorphins, may engender symptoms of physiological dependence. Therefore, some investigators have likened excessive exercising to opioid addiction, and biological studies suggest some overlap between these conditions. However, the epidemiological and clinical data on excessive exercising as a psychiatric disorder are currently relatively modest. No standard criteria for identifying the condition exist, and populations that presumably differ with respect to their frequencies and intensities of exercising do not always differ in the expected manner in terms of problems arising from excessive exercising. In some cases, excessive exercising appears to align more closely with eating and obsessive–compulsive disorders than with substance use disorders. Exercise addiction could benefit from further study, but future research should focus on broad groups of persons who exercise excessively and evaluate common phenomenology, rather than tailoring descriptions to nongeneralizable samples. Much research to date has focused on professional athletes, specific types of athletes, or college student samples. A broader application of this construct is needed to ascertain its public health significance and potential for classification as a psychiatric disorder.

As outlined by Drs. Murray, Gold, and Avena in Chapter 8, excessive eating or food addiction has commonalities with eating disorders, but it also shares some overlap with addictions. Similar to exercising, ingestion of highly palatable foods can release endorphins and dopamine, producing pleasurable sensations. A syndrome that mimics physiological dependence may ensue following regular ingestion of these types of foods, and symptoms of withdrawal may present when ingestion does not occur. Animal laboratory paradigms have shed light on the construct of food addiction, but additional studies directly comparing effects of palatable food to drugs of abuse may clarify similarities and differences between responses to them. In clinical samples, people with "food addiction" express strong cravings for foods, as individuals with substance use disorders do for drugs of abuse. Many of the criteria for substance use disorders apply to excessive eating of foods as well. In fact, the most popularly utilized tool to assess excessive eating, the Yale Food Addiction Scale, adapted the DSM-IV criteria for substance use disorders.

Despite interest in the construct of food addiction, additional clinical research must ascertain whether food addiction is a separate and unique disorder or if it represents a more severe form of other eating disorders. If it is a distinct condition, then more studies must clarify the criteria for classifying it. Some characteristics of food addiction may be distinct from those associated with substance use. Clinicians appear to treat food addiction similar to substance use disorders, but randomized clinical trials must evaluate these interventions systematically to determine whether they confer benefits beyond existing treatments for eating disorders. Some pharmacotherapies may reduce addictive eating behaviors as well. An important next step is to develop and evaluate prevention efforts at individual and societal levels. More than 30% of the U.S. population is now overweight or obese, and many industrialized countries are following this trend, with increasingly large proportions of populations reaching unhealthy weights that result in adverse health consequences. Regardless of whether food addiction is a unique psychiatric disorder, the public health significance of preventing and treating overweight and obesity is paramount.

Finally, a condition of growing interest that has both biological and psychological overlap with addictive disorders is tanning addiction (Chapter 9). Drs. Stapleton, Hillhouse, and Coups review the strong biological evidence that tanning releases endorphins and stimulates dopamine receptors. These two biological effects have clear similarities to those associated with drugs of abuse. Criteria assessing tanning addiction are drawn from those related to substance use disorders. They appear to have construct validity for identifying individuals who tan excessively. Nevertheless, general population studies are lacking, and the extent to which people other than college students engage in excessive tanning behaviors is unknown. It is also unclear whether tanning interferes with important aspects of life functioning and the specific adverse effects it engenders. Still, some persons report that they miss school or work to tan, and tanning has clear adverse negative health effects. Little research to date finds high rates of comorbidity between tanning addiction and substance use or other behavioral addictions, but some research points to it overlapping with body dysmorphic disorder. Thus, similar to many of the putative behavioral addictions, excessive tanning may relate more to psychiatric conditions other than addictions. Although little clinical research is available to guide interventions, some mental health professions are treating persons who tan excessively using approaches for treating substance use disorders. From a public health perspective, increased legislation and regulation of indoor tanning, especially among adolescents, is warranted due to the clear adverse health consequences from tanning.

In summary, many excessive behavior patterns exert harms to individuals and society at large. This book outlines potential behavioral addictions for which there are at least some data related to assessment, prevalence rates, risk and protective factors, neurobiology, and treatment. Some conditions have more data related to biological mechanisms, whereas others have greater evidence related to assessment and treatment. However, none of these conditions has well-established classification criteria with strong evidence of reliability and validity in general population and clinical samples.

In part because of the lack of evidence and consistency in classification, the DSM-5 did not include any of these conditions, but it opened the door for behavioral addictions. By aligning gambling disorder with substance use disorders, it allows for inclusion of other non-substance or behavioral addictions alongside these disorders. However, the DSM-5 cautiously included only one well0established, non-substance or behavioral addiction in the main text—gambling disorder.

The research appendix of the DSM-5 provides the first attempt to standardize classification of Internet gaming disorder. Researchers ultimately may adapt and study these criteria in the context of excessive Internet use for other purposes or behavioral addictions more generally. Caution must be extended, however, because not all conditions share similar phenomenological expressions. Without careful evaluation of the unique clinical expressions and natural courses of these excessive behavior patterns, using a common approach for assessing behavioral addictions may obscure rather than enhance their understanding and treatment.

A broad adaptation of addiction criteria may have more generalized adverse consequences as well. The literature and media are replete with examples of addictions to things such as love, work, chocolate, tango, and even railroad building. Although people can engage in a wide variety of excessive behavioral patterns, certainly not all are psychiatric disorders. Aligning expressions of these behavior patterns with serious mental health disorders will detract from the field of psychiatry overall.

As clinicians and researchers gain greater awareness and understanding of conditions such as Internet gaming disorder, Internet addiction, sex addiction or hypersexuality, shopping addiction, exercise addiction, food addiction, and tanning addiction, they must consider both the similarities and unique nature of expression of these conditions relative to substance use and gambling disorders. They should also consider their overlap and distinctions from other closely aligned conditions, such as eating disorders, sexual disorders, and obsessive–compulsive or impulse control disorders.

Whether conditions that result in clinically significant harms are classified as behavioral addictions or under another rubric is less important than recognizing the condition as a psychiatric disorder. Only with concentrated efforts toward consistent and valid classification will individuals suffering from these conditions benefit from appropriate assessment and treatment. Systematic research on the expression, clinical course, risk factors, family history, neurobiology, and treatment of these conditions will further the field of psychiatry and improve the quality of lives of people who develop these and related problems. The chapters in this book review the state of the science in these areas, and they should guide future research to realize this greater goal.

REFERENCES

American Psychiatric Association, 2013. *Diagnostic and statistical manual of mental disorders* (5th ed.). Washington, DC: American Psychiatric Association.
Lesieur, H.R., Blume, S.B., 1987. The South Oaks Gambling Screen (SOGS): A new instrument for the identification of pathological gamblers. Am J Psychiatry. 144, 1184–1188.

Page numbers followed by *t* or *b* indicate tables or boxes, respectively. Numbers followed by n indicate notes.